I0095173

Dr. Douglass'

Complete Guide to

BETTER VISION

William Campbell Douglass II, MD

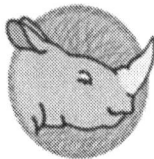

Rhino Publishing, S.A.
Panama City
Republic of Panama

Dr. Douglass'
Complete Guide to
BETTER
VISION

Copyright © 1997, 2003
by
William Campbell Douglass II, MD

All rights reserved. Copyright under Berne Copyright Convention, Universal Copyright Convention, and Pan-American Copyright Convention. No part of this book may be reproduced, stored in a retrieval system, or transmitted in any form, or by any means, electronic, mechanical, photocopying, recording or otherwise, without prior written permission of the publisher and author.

ISBN 9962-636-18-3

Cover illustration by

Alex Manyoma (alex@3dcity.com)

Please, visit Rhino's website for other publications from
Dr. William Campbell Douglass
www.rhinopublish.com

Dr. Douglass' "Real Health" alternative medical newsletter is available at www.realhealthnews.com

RHINO PUBLISHING, S.A.
World Trade Center
Panama, Republic of Panama

Voicemail/Fax
International: + 416-352-5126
North America: 888-317-6767

Table of Contents

Introduction

Eyes.

They are two of our most precious assets. And everybody wants them to work perfectly. I know I do.

When they don't, life becomes proportionally more difficult to the degree that they don't work.

Thanks to modern technology, though, much can be done to help the weaker and diseased eye.

But is modern technology the end-all of eye treatment? I hardly think so. People have been dealing with eye problems since the earliest days of his creation, and eye glasses, contacts, and laser surgery are all relatively new.

Now, don't get me wrong. Many of the latest advances in eye treatment are absolutely marvelous and we'll be discussing some of those in this report. I also don't think our ancestors had all the answers. But I'm not a throw-the-baby-out-with-the-bath-water person. In fact, one of my motto's is: "If it works for you, use it."

As a result, I know a lot of you will read only the sections of this report that deal with your specific problems. That's fine. But let me encourage you to read the entire manuscript. Why? Because if you don't have a particular eye problem now, there's a good chance you probably will somewhere down the road. If you decided to wait until you have the problem, it may be too late. And a little prevention goes a long way.

Our eyesight will deteriorate with age: Decreased visual acuity and the need for glasses, cataracts, and eventually macular degeneration are an inevitable part of the aging process in most people. That isn't a pleasant thought, but it is reality. Although some people reach 80 with remarkably good eyesight.

We don't know if this is genetic good luck or from healthy living. I suspect it's from choosing the right parents, but I am by no means sure about this. I think most ophthalmologists would say it is 99 percent genetics. They may be right. Whatever the answer, and maybe it's a combination of both, our aim is to slow the deterioration process and enable you to read the newspaper and your Bible — Old or New Testament — on the last day of your life in the year 20_.

That's why I decided to write a report about eyesight and what can be done to improve it naturally. But I've also included information about how the eye works, brief descriptions of various common eye conditions, traditional remedies to eye problems, and a few simple suggestions that may help you maintain your eyesight for years to come.

So even if you don't read this report in its entirety now, do yourself a favor and at least skim the topics and subheads. Then file it somewhere for "future reference" — the basic information will not change much.

The Eye Doctor

I usually tell my subscribers to stay away from doctors because they often make you sicker than you were before you went to his office. But my advice for seeing the eye doctor is a little different. I agree that it's a good idea to have your eyes checked even if you have no symptoms. Once examined, you will have a reference point for your visual acuity to which you can compare progress or lack thereof.

However, if your doctor tells you to take some course of action, whether it be surgery or buying corrective lenses, tell him you must think about it for a few weeks (or months, if it's not an emergency-type situation) before submitting to his advice. That will give you time to see if there are alternatives you can try first. A change in diet, a few specific eye exercises, the use of a few herbs, and the avoidance of particular food additives can go a long way to helping you maintain and even improve your sight. Too many of us blindly follow the advice of our doctors, allowing them to take our ignorance to the bank.

Let me add here that most eye doctors are honorable men, and proud of their profession. But, as in any field, there are some who are more interested in the cash than your cataracts — beware of these "cataract cowboys."

One caveat: If you notice a sudden decline in your eyesight, or sudden pain in an eye, please see your doctor. Eye problems can often be averted by quick action. This report should give you enough information to help you make an informed decision, but please, if you encounter a sudden decline in eyesight, a red eye or eye pain, follow this advice. After all, you will have only two eyes in your entire life; it is not likely that an eye transplant is in your future.

Optometrists, Ophthalmologists, and Opticians

But I am often asked: "Should I see an optometrist, an ophthalmologist, an optician, or my friendly eye-care professional at K-Mart? Vision-care providers go by different titles and the services they provide vary from state to state and country to country. Here's a quick summary of who does what:

The Optometrist has the degree Doctor of Optometry (O.D.) and is a primary vision-care specialist. He has completed four years of college and a two-year course in optometry.

An optometrist can examine your eyes and related structures for health and vision disorders and treat vision problems with spectacle and contact lenses and exercises. In all but nine states, optometrists dispense eyeglasses and contact lenses.

Doctors of Optometry also may treat certain eye diseases. The type of eye diseases they may medically treat vary from state to state.

The Ophthalmologist has the degree Doctor of Medicine (M.D.) and is a primary and secondary, medical/surgical eye-care provider. He has completed four years of college, four years of medical school, and three years or more of residency and internship relating to the diagnosis and treatment, including surgery, of diseases of the eye. Some ophthalmologists specialize in treating very specific eye problems. These include the treatment of retinal and corneal diseases.

Ophthalmologists may also perform intricate surgical procedures including cataract removal and crystalline lens transplants and various repairs and therapies utilizing lasers. In some locales, they also provide vision examinations and may dispense contact lenses and eyeglasses.

The services you may receive from an ophthalmologist or optometrist may be nearly identical or considerably different and limited in scope. This would depend on where the practice is located and what specialties the doctor chooses to provide. As the United States moves toward managed care systems, (and perhaps in the future universal, "accessible" national health care) the optometrist's role seems to be moving toward one of primary-care provider. Ophthalmologists, then, become specialists who deal with more involved medical and surgical treatments.

There are eye doctors in both fields who take exception to these alterations and delineations of their roles in the health care system. For now, you will have to inquire as to the level of eye care provided by these practitioners. *When in doubt, go to an ophthalmologist.*

The optician is a person who has trained in the skills necessary to grind and shape glass and plastic materials to the optical powers as prescribed by an O.D. or M.D. Education consists of trade school and apprenticeship. An optician may hold various certifications and licenses, which vary by state and county of practice. An optician is also the person who operates a facility that dispenses eyeglasses and other accessories. In some states and countries, they may also dispense contact lenses as prescribed by a doctor. In the United States and most elsewhere, they cannot examine the eyes.

Basic Eye Problems and How to Deal With Them

There are basically four common visual refractive disorders of the eye. They are called myopia (near-sightedness), hyperopia (farsightedness), presbyopia, and astigmatism. If you wear glasses, you've undoubtedly heard of one or more of these conditions.

When you get a prescription from your eye doctor for one of these disorders, you'll notice several numbers. These numbers represent units of measure called 'diopters,' which are the amount of correction needed in corrective lenses to normalize vision. The more nearsighted or farsighted you are, the higher your prescription in diopters.

Your prescription will look something like this: -5.00/ -1.25 x 175.

The first number identifies your degree of nearsightedness or farsightedness. The (-) sign indicates you are nearsighted, the (+) sign indicates you are farsighted.

The second number identifies your degree of astigmatism. The sign can be either plus or minus.

And the third number is the axis, which indicates the direction of your astigmatism.

Called "shortsighted," or "nearsighted," **myopia** is the inability to see distant objects clearly. The optical problem is that the image produced by the eye focuses just short of (in front of) the retina, leaving a blurred image to fall on the retina. More than 70 million people in North America are nearsighted. Myopia occurs when an eye is too long for the cornea's curvature. Thus light rays entering the eye do not come to a sharp focus on the retina at the back of the eye.

The table below shows the categories of severity for myopia:

Mild Myopia	<-3.00 diopters
Moderate Myopia	-3.00 to -6.00 diopters
Severe Myopia	-6.00 to -9.00 diopters
Extreme Myopia	>-9.00 diopters

Almost everyone feels that their myopia is severe, because of how dependent they are on glasses and contact lenses. However, only one in ten myopic people are actually in the severe and extreme categories.

Astigmatism is the condition where a point focus cannot be formed on the retina. The refraction of light is unequal in different meridians. This means lines in one direction may be blurred while others are not. Astigmatics often report double vision (diplopia) or even multiple images (polyplopia) in both eyes or even a single eye.

Conventional optometry treats astigmatism through the prescription of lenses. "Behavioral optometry" regards astigmatism as correctable with vision therapy. In certain cases, I believe it can be corrected by the proper exercises.

Elliot Forrest O.D. found a relationship between head movement, posture, and visual scanning. If you use a computer or read a lot then you will tend to scan from along the horizontal meridian and neglect the vertical meridian, with a resultant astigmatism in that meridian. I don't find it easy to accept this theory of acquired astigmatism.

Some say that astigmatism may also result from a twisting of the spine, pelvis, or neck.

Astigmatism is also measured in diopters. Of all myopic people, 50 percent or more have astigmatism as well. Most of these people have corrections of less than 1 diopter. The table below shows the categories of severity for astigmatism:

Mild Astigmatism:	< 1.00 diopters
Moderate Astigmatism	1.00 to 2.00 diopters
Severe Astigmatism	2.00 to 3.00 diopters
Extreme Astigmatism	> 3.00 diopters

Hyperopia is the medical term for "farsightedness." It occurs when an eye is too short for the cornea's curvature. Light rays entering the eye focus behind the retina and, as a result, a blurred image is produced. Farsighted individuals, however, can use their focusing muscles to "pull" the image forward onto the retina. In a young person with severe hyperopia, or once presbyopia (see next paragraph) sets in around age 45, distant objects are seen more clearly than near objects.

Presbyopia is the normal process of aging, where the natural lens of the eye loses some of the flexibility that characterizes a younger eye. Everyone experiences presbyopia; some sooner, some later. Because of this normal process, farsighted people begin to wear bifocals in their 40s.

The crystalline lens, located inside your eye and just behind the pupil, is responsible for adjusting the focus from a distance point to a near point. The tiny ciliary muscle pulls and pushes on the lens altering it's curvature, thereby changing it's focal power. As we age, the lens becomes less flexible and the ciliary muscle becomes less powerful. This is a slow process, starting during the third decade of life and becoming symptomatic by age 45 or 50.

The time in which this becomes a problem varies considerably. The eyes, like many other parts of the human body, age on different schedules for different people. At what age one would notice the effects of presbyopia depends upon not only the physiologic aging of the eye, but also on the demands placed on the vision system. However, using your eyes does not make the situation worse, and in fact may delay the onset of acute symptoms. This is one example of the "use it or loose it" principal. As you'll see in a moment, relaxation of the eyes is vital.

The traditional approach for treating presbyopia is simply to use near or reading glasses. If you need prescription lenses for distance as well, bifocal lenses may be in order. Near eyeglasses provide the degree of focusing no longer provided by your crystalline lens. There are also multi-focal contact lenses and monovision contact lenses. Exercising the ciliary muscle is sometimes helpful and nutrition plays a role.

The exercises are most effective for people who are just beginning to have difficulties focusing up close.

Step 1: "Tromboning": Start by holding an object with relatively small reading print, such as a business card, at arm's distance away from your eyes. Make sure that the object is located in the mid-line centered with your nose and not favoring either eye. It should also be located slightly below eye level. Begin by focusing on the card and slowly bring it closer to your eyes. A rate of movement about one inch (2.5cm) per second is correct. At a certain point the image will begin to blur. Stop here and concentrate and try to clear the image for two seconds. Now reverse the process and push the card away from your eyes. When you reach the limit of your arm's length, look at a distance object at least 20 feet (6m) away. Immediately return your attention and focus to the near card and repeat the process of bringing it closer to your eyes. Repeat this process ten times.

Step 2: "Straddling the blur point push ups": Bring the near object in to the point of just noticeable blur. While concentrating to keep it in focus, very slowly bring it closer to the point of increased blur. Now strongly make an effort to clear the image. You may notice that your peripheral vision appears to dim slightly. This is because the extraordinary effort you are putting forth to focus is also causing your iris and pupil to constrict, thereby reducing the total amount of light entering your eye. This is good feedback indicating you are making maximum effort to focus. Now push the near object back away to the point of clear vision and then bring it closer in to the point of blur and, again, really concentrate to clear the blur. Repeat ten times. Now repeat step 1, tromboning for ten more times.

That's it. You should do this exercises two or three times per day. Results are often apparent within a few days and maximum benefit is achieved within about a month.

How do you know if the exercises are working? Before beginning each session, measure your near point at which the object begins to blur and at which it is definitely blurred, even with maximum effort to prevent the blurring. Use a measuring stick and measure from a point at the bridge of your nose. As days pass, you should notice that the near point of blur becomes closer to your eyes. If you see no change within one week, you will not likely be successful. If you do see improvement, continue the exercise program until you no longer can record any additional benefit.

Floaters

The small specks or "bugs" that many people see moving in their field of vision are called floaters. They are frequently visible when looking at a plain background, such as a blank wall or blue sky and in bright light. Floaters were described long ago, in Roman times, as flying flies *(muscae volitantes)*.

Most ophthalmologists would describe floaters as small clumps of gel that form in the vitreous, the clear jelly-like fluid that fills the inside cavity of the eye. Although they appear to be in front of the eye, they are actually floating in the fluid inside the eye and are seen as shadows by the retina (the light-sensing inner layer of the eye).

However, Dr. William Bates argued back in the first half of this century that the vast majority of floaters are not pieces of debris floating around in the eye, but are simply an illusion resulting from mental strain. In his book, *Better Eyesight Without Glasses* (Henry Holt, 1981), Dr. Bates contends, "The specks are never seen, in other words, except when the eyes and mind are under a strain, and they always disappear when the strain is relieved."

Dr. Bates is the most famous advocate of natural exercise for eye care and his book is a classic — although optometrists passionately disagree. As you can see, his words fly in the face of almost all the current literature on floaters. According to Bates, "Some have attributed [floaters] to the presence of floating specks — dead cells or the debris of cells — in the vitreous humor.... Similar specks on the surface of the cornea have also been held responsible for them. It has even been surmised that they might be caused by the passage of tears over the cornea.

"They are so common in myopia that they have been supposed to be one of the symptoms of this condition, although they occur also with other errors of refraction as well as in eyes otherwise normal. They have been attributed to disturbances of the circulation, the digestion, and the kidneys, and because so many insane people have them, they have been thought to be an evidence of incipient insanity. The patent-medicine business has thrived upon them, and it would be difficult to estimate the amount of mental torture they have caused...."

The appearance of floaters, whether in the form of little dots, circles, lines, or cobwebs, may cause much concern, especially if they develop suddenly. However, they are usually of little importance, representing the aging process in some, but from stress in most.

Floaters may sometimes interfere with clear vision, often when reading, and can be quite annoying. If a floater appears directly in your line of vision, the best thing to do is to move your eye around, which will cause the inside fluid to swirl and allow the floater to move out of the way. We are most accustomed to moving our eyes back and forth, but looking up and down will cause different currents within the eye and may be more effective in getting the floaters out of the way.

The size and shape of the spots vary among individuals. Some are only slightly noticeable, while others may be quite disturbing when they drift in the field of vision, especially if it looks like a blackbird just flew across the room. Often they appear as dust-like particles, cobwebs, or thread-like strands. They can also appear as dim or dark areas, or showers of brilliant crystals. Since spots move as the eye moves, they dart away when the patient tries to look directly at them.

So how do we get rid of these floaters? The answer is definitely not surgery! The best remedy I know of is Dr. Bates' prescription to *relax*. Here's what Bates says about it:

"Fortunately all persons are able to relax under certain conditions at will. In all uncomplicated errors of refraction, the strain to see can be relieved, temporarily, by having the patient look at a blank wall without trying to see. To secure permanent relaxation sometimes requires considerable time and much ingenuity. The same method cannot be used with everyone. The ways in which people strain to see are infinite, and methods used to relieve the strain must be almost equally varied. Whatever the method that brings most relief, however, the end is always the same, namely, relaxation. By constant repetition and frequent demonstration and by all means possible, the fact must be stressed that perfect sight can be obtained only by relaxation."

One Method of Relaxation

Here's a very brief summary of Dr. Bates' relaxation methods. As Bates said, there is more than one way to relax, and each person's methods can vary. But I think his method, if followed precisely, is the best way to go. You'll have to read the book to understand the value of his entire process.

1. Close your eyes. While doing this, think of something agreeable.

2. Cover your eyes — called "palming." If you cover your eyes so as to exclude all light, the eyes will be able to achieve a greater degree of relaxation. Cover both eyes with the palms of your hands, your fingers crossed on your forehead. Note: In order to be successful, you must be able to relax while palming. Some people cannot do this, and palming becomes counterproductive. The blacker the field you see, the more relaxed you are. But if you "try" to see black, this may cause more strain. Don't try to see black: It is better to imagine a concrete, familiar object or scene.

3. Observe the swing of things. As you move your gaze from one point to another, things seen should move in the opposite direction. For example, if you look at the upper left corner of the letter "H" and then shift your gaze to the lower left corner, the "H" should appear to move, or "swing" up. If it doesn't, this is a sign of strain. There are a variety of exercises to practice the swing. You can gently swing your whole body to the left and to the right, and watch a distant tree swing to the right and to the left, you can move just your head, or just your eyes. The better the vision, the shorter the swing can be made to be.

4. Use your imagination. By seeing things with your mind's eye, and remembering them in precise detail, you in-

crease your ability to see actual objects better. The perfect memory of any sensation can be produced only when one is free of strain.

5. Catch those flashes. When your eyes finally achieve a state of relaxation through swinging or palming, you will see a "clear flash"; paradoxically, the sight of everything in focus is such a surprise that it causes strain, and the blur returns. So before the clear picture blurs out, close your eyes and remember the image in its full sharpness and clarity.

6. Keep your vision centered. When you regard an object, only one small part should be seen best. This is because only the center of the retina — the fovea — has the best vision for detail. Farther away from the fovea, the retinal receptors get progressively less able to pick up fine detail. Therefore, trying to catch all the detail with all of your retina at once causes strain because it cannot be done. Instead of staring at the entirety of an image, restrict your attention to the smallest area that you can.

7. Enjoy the sun. Get out into the open and enjoy every sunny day. It is especially relaxing and stimulating to the eyes if you close your eyes and let the sun shine onto your lids as you sway back and forth.

8. Practice with a test card. Keep an eye chart on the wall. To practice, stand from 10-20 feet away, and read the smallest line that you can without straining. Then look at one of the letters on that line and close your eyes. Remember that letter — go over every detail in your mind; shift from part to part, from curve to corner, and so on. When you open your eyes, you will see not only that letter better, but also the one below it. If you find yourself staring at the letters, which results in the line becoming blurred as soon as it comes into focus, it is best to close the eyes before this can happen. When you open them, shift to another letter on the same line. If you close your eyes for each letter, you will become able to read the whole line. Practice every day for five minutes or more and record your progress.

Does this work? I don't know and the only way an individual can know is to try it. Dr. Bates' book is so insightful, that I heartily recommend it for anyone suffering from *minor* eye problems. In fact, his methods should always be tried before you submit to any corrective lenses or surgery. You can order the book from your local bookstore. You'll need to provide the salesperson with the publisher's name and the book's ISBN (Henry Holt, 0-8050-0241-3). I got my copy for under $10 — a lot less than a trip to the eye doctor.

Can vision actually be improved?

Some of you may be skeptical, but the answer is yes. In many cases, improvements are possible. Conditions like myopia, astigmatism, and hyperopia can often be corrected significantly, depending on the individual condition, motivation, and the inherent flexibility of the visual system.

The U.S. Air Force and many commercial airlines have programs training pilots with normal vision to super normal sight. Olympic athletes, including the U.S. volleyball and field hockey teams, frequently work to improve their sight to beyond normal. Other athletes who do so include tennis champion Virginia Wade, the Dallas Cowboys, New York Yankees, and professional golfer Val Skinner. The Connecticut state police have regular vision improvement training.

The key to improving your eyesight is taking a small amount of time each day to care for your eyes. Just as you exercise to keep your body in shape and read to keep your mind in shape, it's necessary to do a few simple things to help maintain your vision. And in some cases, it's simply a matter of replacing new vision habits with old, bad habits.

Glasses are a necessary evil for many of us

Unfortunately, in many cases, glasses are necessary, no doubt. In others, however, glasses and contact lens worsen sight.

Glass and plastic lenses in spectacles and contact lenses interfere with the transmission of light. Color is always more intense when seem with the naked eye than with any lens. It can be argued that since color is a major part of the perception of form it follows that in small to medium sight defects, form is not as well perceived with glasses.

Secondly, its possible that glasses actually aggravate the eye, by constantly maintaining a degree of refractive error, which otherwise would not be there. This too is a necessary evil in most cases.

Unless your glasses are quartz crystal, which isn't likely, you are not receiving the full spectrum of light and may have what Dr. John Ott has called "light-deficiency disease." Over a period of years this may affect your health.

The strong concave glasses required by myopes of high degree make all objects seem much smaller than they really are, while convex glasses enlarge them. Patients with a degree of astigmatism can suffer some very disagreeable sensations when they put on glasses. Usually these difficulties are overcome, but sometimes they are not. And those who do overcome them during the day, may never succeed in getting used to them at night.

All glasses constrict the field of vision to a greater or lesser degree. Often glasses cause annoying nerve symptoms, such as dizziness and headache, and the frames also interfere with peripheral vision. But in spite of some drawbacks, half the world would be essentially incapacitated without glasses. In fact, in many Third World countries millions of the elderly are nonfunctioning because *they can't see.*

Many Russian civilians during World War II were known to wear negative diopter lenses for several days prior to visual examinations in compulsory enlistments in order to fail the eye test. I don't know if the story is true. Why wouldn't a young Russian boy want to go to the Western front in minus 40-degree weather to be shot at by the Germans? I suspect these draft evaders were kidding themselves — a hundred-dollar bribe would have been far more effective.

Glasses do not give you "perfect vision." Refraction is continually changing from day to day, from hour to hour, and from minute to minute (a fact that is easily verified by personal observation). Thus the completely accurate fitting of glasses or contacts is impossible.

Reflections of strong light from eyeglasses are often very annoying, and in the street may be very dangerous. Expensive coatings are needed to reduce these effects. In so doing, they reduce the brightness of colors. These coatings also require special cloths to clean, and they scratch easily requiring a hardness coating.

Many people have great difficulties with glasses because of the activity of their lives. A high-activity lifestyle can lead to broken lenses, or it could throw them out of focus, particularly in the case of eyeglasses worn for astigmatism.

Contact lenses are difficult to clean and maintain. They are often dropped and, if not scrupulously cleaned, can lead to various eye infections. Astigmatism is often corrected poorly, due to the lens rotating on the eye. Even the most permeable contacts deprive the eye of oxygen and capillaries may extend into the cornea as a result. Extended wear lenses are notorious for causing infections and complications.

The progression of myopia, shortsightedness, often means that a perfect prescription is quickly inadequate and the patient spends most of his time with a noticeable amount of refractive error. In fact, most optometrists under-correct myopia to begin with. Contrary to popular belief, 20/20 vision does not mean 100 percent of the human visual potential, but the average acuity of people living during the time the standard was established.

The lenses generally prescribed by classical optometrists are called compensating lenses, in that they only compensate for refractive errors and have no therapeutic value. In a progressive hyperopic, the lenses quickly become a total addiction. This is not the optometrists' fault; it's just the way it is. The eye doctor is giving you a crutch for a failing system. I have a friend who is so vain at age 78, and so convinced that his glasses will make him "dependant" on them (at least that's what he says is his excuse for not wearing them) that I no longer hand him anything to read — he never has his glasses.

But the sad truth is that many of us wouldn't be able to see at all without glasses. It's definitely a Catch-22 situation, but I'm sure you'd agree that using glasses is the better option.

The Dry Eye

Dry Eye Syndrome, and the symptoms associated with it, is one of most common problems reported to eye doctors.

The clinically dry eye is considered to be an ocular surface disease associated with "tear film" deficiencies or a poorly functioning tear film. Symptoms include: burning, stinging, a gritty sandy feeling, a foreign body sensation (feels like something stuck under the eye lid), itching, and often excessive tearing. Sometimes there are strands of stringy mucous present as well.

A common questions is: How can I have dry eye syndrome if one of my symptoms is watering eyes? This will be explained below.

The treatment of the dry eye focuses on providing substitute artificial tears and lubrication aimed at increasing and enhancing the existing tear production, obstructing the tear outflow to maximize tear contact time with the cornea and other eye tissues, and treatment of the underlying cause if it can be determined.

This last issue is quite important. Certain tear film deficiencies are related to systemic diseases, medications and other drugs, and environmental causes. Systemic diseases that may be associated with the clinically dry eye include: Sjorgen's syndrome, thyroid dysfunction, diminished estrogen production, certain autoimmune disorders, Bell's palsy, myasthenia gravis, and other neurological disorders affecting lid closure and tear production.

Drugs and medications are also an issue. Alcohol, and to some degree caffeine, have a dehydrating effect on body fluids in general, smoke from tobacco products are irritants that cause an over production of lacrimal tears resulting in a drying effect (see below).

There are numerous medications that affect tear production. These include: antianxiety and antidepression agents, medicines for hypertension, antihistamines, decongestants, and other medications.

Environmental causes include: air-conditioning and heating, chemical vapors and smoke, and intensive and prolonged near vision tasks. The reason why people engaged in near-vision tasks experience dry eye symptoms is because their blink rate decreases and this allows the tear film to dehydrate more rapidly. (See the section on computers and eyestrain, page 21.)

It is highly recommended that people who experience dry-eye symptoms seek diagnosis and management from an eye doctor. It is often appropriate to address the underlying cause along with, and sometimes prior to, providing symptomatic relief. Do consult with your eye doctor before beginning treatment. Otherwise, you may do more harm than good.

The tear system

To understand the cause of the symptoms and treatments, it is useful to know how the tear film works. Scientifically called the "pre-corneal tear film multilayer structure," the tears have a number of specific functions:

1. Provide water to maintain the hydration of the cornea and carry oxygen and nutritional support.
2. Carry antibacterial and antiviral cells to protect the exposed structures of the eye from infection.
3. Carry off debris so it does not damage the sensitive tissue of the eye.
4. Provide lubrication between the inside of the lids and the cornea.

The tear film is actually composed of three separate films:
* a layer of mucus, which lies against the eyeball
* a layer of water, which is the middle layer
* a layer of oil, which covers the other two.

There are a number of glands (and the associated duct systems) that produce these components. They reside in the eyelids and in a special gland called the lacrimal gland at the inner side of each eyeball. In a properly functioning system, the three elements are produced in perfect balance, mixed, and distributed across the eyeball with every blink. You should be unaware of the tear film's existence. Then again, something might happen to disrupt this balance and any or all of the previously discussed symptoms occur.

When the oil or mucus layer is disrupted, our bodies try to compensate in the simplest manner — produce more tears. The problem is that the tears that are produced quickly upon demand are lacrimal tears, consisting mostly of just water and salt. The newly dispensed watery tears simply run off the now destablized tear film. The eyes get dry, red, and irritated. The resulting dry spots on the cornea result in more discomfort, which causes more lacrimal tearing, which further destablizes the tear film, etc. An interesting note: When we cry, we are producing excessive lacrimal tears that tend to destabilize the tear film causing a dry eye, hence the red, irritated look after crying.

Treating the dry eye

To treat dry eye, most eye doctors use artificial tear replacement drops, of which there are a number of brands and formulations. The primary differences between the products are: preserved or non-preserved, the level of viscosity (thickness), and the degree of lubrication (slipperiness) of the agents.

Depending upon the severity of tear film dysfunction and symptoms, the dry eye is treated by frequent and proper instillation of the appropriate artificial tear replacement drops. A list of currently available drops follows.

"Frequent" means every two hours. Proper application requires the placement of one drop into the sack created when you gently pull the lower lid out and away from the eyeball. You then close the eyes slowly, open and blink once (to mix the drop with the natural tears) and then close the eyes for 30 seconds. This allows the artificial tears to form temporary attachments to the ocular surface, prolonging the beneficial effects.

This therapy is continued for three to five days (up to two weeks if there are severe symptoms), then the frequency is diminished — using the drops every fours hours, then every six hours over the next week or so. You will find there is a certain frequency of administering the drops that maintains comfort. Sometimes it is possible to slowly taper off the artificial tears. If the underlying cause is mitigated, the use of tear replacements may stabilize the tear layer situation, allowing the body to resume normal tear film production.

It is not appropriate to prescribe tear-replacement drops for use "as needed" or desired. By the time the patient experiences dry-eye symptoms, the tear film has already destabilized, the corneal surface has been impacted and the syndrome has been established. Proper treatment is designed to prevent this situation from occurring by intervening early and encouraging the body to create a more normal environment.

List of available artificial tears

When choosing a tear replacement drop, many doctors prefer to use non-preserved products as the preservatives themselves can exacerbate the symptoms. The downside of preservative-free products is their limited shelf life, single use or limited use containers, and the possibility of contamination from misuse. (The tip of the dropper must not contact the eye or fingers.) Users must not allow the packaging to be exposed to extremes of heat and cold. Lanolin-free ointments are preferable for those with allergy to wool.

For your convenience, I've listed the names of eye drops you'll find in your local drug store. (All are available over-the-counter, no prescription required.) For most people with mild to moderate dry eye syndrome, these should work without any side effects. However, I personally don't like these preparations, as frequent use can cause chronic eye irritation. As a result, I've provided an alternative at the end of this section that you should seriously consider using if you suffer from dry eye.

Non-preserved products

Viva Drops (Vision Pharmaceuticals) contains vitamin A, but it is not marketed as therapeutic. It is reported as very effective, but no formal double-blind, controlled studies have been published. Many patients find this to be one of the best drops for mild to moderate dry-eye syndrome.

Tears Naturale Free (Alcon) is well-tolerated and usable for mild to moderate dry eye.

OcuCoat PF (Storz) is best suited for severe dry eyes and prior to retiring. They may blur vision.

Hypotears PF (lolab) is an old standby in newer preservative-free formulation.

Refresh Plus (Allergan) is also an old standby, well- tolerated and effective, especially in less severe dry eyes.

Bion Tears (Alcon) is a newer product very well tolerated and effective for moderately severe dry eyes. Very similar to Tears Natural Free.

Similasan 1 (Similasan) is a homeopathic and herbal formulation drop, very soothing and effective in mild dry eye syndrome.

Celluvisc (Allergan) is used primarily for severe dry eyes and for use prior to retiring. It may blur vision. This is a more concentrated version of Refresh Plus.

Refresh PM (Allergan) ointment is designed for use prior to retiring. It is for severe dry eyes.

DuaTears Naturale (Alcon) is similar to Refresh PM for severe dry eyes.

Hypotears Ointment (Ciba) lanolin free, for severe dry eyes.

Duolube Ointment lanolin free, for severe dry eyes.

Preserved products

Tears Naturale II solution, contains polyquad **Tears Plus** solution, contains chlorbutanol **Aquasite** (Ciba) A newer, advanced agent for severe dry eyes, contains EDTA.

OcuCoat solution, contains benzalkonium chloride **Lacrilube** ointment

The alternative

The easiest eyewash for regular use that I've been able to find is in *Earl Mindell's Herb Bible* (Simon & Schuster, 1992). Mindell writes: "If you need to use an eyewash, try eyebright. Mix two tablespoons of the herb in 16 ounces hot water. Let cool. Strain. Use a small cup to pour mixture into each eye, or apply to each eye with a clean cotton ball. (Do not use the same cotton ball for both eyes, as this may spread the infection.)"

I think you'll be amazed at how well this herb works.

Computers and eyestrain

I've stuck this section in right here because computer users are some of the worst sufferers of dry eye. If you are not a computer user, you may want to skip this section.

Americans are developing eye problems at an earlier age. This may be, in part, because of food additives we consume (aspartame being one of the worst for your eyes), but a large reason for these earlier ocular problems may be related to our use of computers. I should know: After working on a small laptop computer for seven years, I've seen a noticeable decline in my ability to read small print — particularly late in the evening. (Couldn't be my age, could it?) If you are a computer user, you may experience computer-related eye strain, tired eyes, and maybe more serious problems.

What to do

Here's what can you do to maximize your body's efficiency at using your eyes:

Control your workspace

1. Adjust the distance between you and the monitor.

For most people, there is a distance somewhere between 56 cm (22") and 91 cm (36") that is most comfortable for the vision system. Try positioning the monitor at a given distance and experience that difference for at least 20 minutes. Move the monitor further out in two-inch increments and repeat until you find the place that feels best for your eyes.

2. Adjust the screen image size

As the monitor is moved further from the eyes, a larger image size is often required. There is, unfortunately, a point of diminishing returns. As you increase the image size, you decrease the total amount of information observed on the screen, which may make your work more difficult.

3. Adjust the monitor's horizontal position.

A monitor at 60 cm should be located as follows: Measure a line from the top of the screen to a point on the center of your forehead between your eyes. The screen should be slightly below the horizontal, creating an angle of about 5-10 degrees, although some people are comfortable with viewing a screen as much as 20 degrees below the horizontal, this depends upon the size of your face and the size of monitor. This angle decreases as the distance from the eyes increases, and vice versa.

4. Adjust brightness and contrast.

Generally, the higher the contrast relative to the brightness is best. Setting the monitor at high contrast and medium brightness is best for most people.

5. Screen color.

Black on white is usually best, as this creates the highest contrast. People with certain visual deficits, however, will find amber or green background screens with white images more comfortable.

6. Ambient lighting.

This is a common and often overlooked problem. Some light in your working environment is critical for viewer comfort, Fluorescent lights create additional screen glare and conflicting flicker. Standard fluorescent lights flicker at 60 hertz. Combine that with a monitor flickering at 60 hertz and you can have trouble.

Two ways around this problem is to use electronic ballast fluorescent (much higher flicker frequency), incandescent lighting, and/or monitors with higher refresh/flicker rates. Natural lighting from outdoor sunshine is, obviously, the best option. North light is always best as any artist or diamond grader will tell you.

7. As cool-white fluorescent tubes are color skewed toward the blue end of the spectrum, eyeglass lenses or screen filters with a 10 percent pink/rose tint can offset and neutralize this effect.

Finally, there is the issue of image stability on the monitor. The easiest-on-the-eyes monitors have the most stable images. LCD screens do not flicker and are quite stable, but unless you have a high resolution screen with high pixel count, the line/edge resolution, lacking in any event, becomes more of an issue than the flicker. Conversely, a CRT monitor with a super-high refresh rate at low pixel count is likewise a poor combination. Most of the better screens will offer high-speed multiscan, interlace/non-interlace options, 75 + hertz refresh rates and high pixel counts. And they cost a thousand dollars and more! If you're setting up a new business or home system and you are going to be spending a lot of time in front of the monitor, invest heavily in the very best. Your eyes deserve it.

8. Rest your eyes periodically:

Take breaks at least every 10 minutes. A break is defined as looking away from the screen to re-focus on a distance (6m + distant) object for a few seconds. Every 20 minutes, get up, stretch your back and neck, and look around. Move your eyes and move your body, change your position.

9. Watch out for dry eyes!

When you look at the computer monitor, there is a natural tendency toward a reduced blink rate. The less you blink, the more likely you are to experience dry-eye symptoms of burning, sand-in-the-eye, heavy lids, etc. You can use tear replacement drops, but being aware of the need to blink is the real fix. The normal blink rate averages 12 times per minute. Computer users usually blink five times per minute. The longer the eye remains open between blinks, the more likely the cornea is to dehydrate, burn, or ache. Then, finally, you blink. But the damage, although minor and easily repaired, is already done. Your eyes sting, burn, and feel miserable. You tear, feel better, then start the process all over again. Eventually, the disruption to the corneal tissue causes a blurred image to go along with the other symptoms. You stop work, fall asleep, and your body fixes the insult.

Special glasses

There is no easy rule of thumb with regard to vision correction, but here's a summary of the related issues:

* If you don't normally require vision correction, computer eyeglasses with low power-plus lenses and sometimes a light tint is often helpful. The color of the tint depends upon the screen background color, ambient room lighting, and your prescription.

* If you use a vision correction for myopia (near-sightedness), a reduced prescription is often recommended, designed for the near working distance. Just taking off your eyeglasses or contacts for near work is generally not a good idea, with some exceptions. (The demand to focus is reduced, but the need to align the eyes is not and a conflict could result.)

* If you use a vision correction of hyperopia (farsightedness) or if you are farsighted and do not generally use eyeglasses, the extra demands of computer use often require a specific vision correction to deal with the specific demands on the vision system.

* If you have astigmatism, it is often very important to have this optical error fully corrected.

24

All You Need to Know
About Cataracts

When it comes to eye problems, I think I get more letters asking about cataracts and cataract surgery than any other problem. And I can definitely understand the concern — I wouldn't want someone operating on my eye unless it was absolutely necessary.

Well, unfortunately, many cases of cataract problems do require surgery. But that's the bad news. There is also some good news, as you'll see in a moment. Because there are so many questions about cataract surgery, I'll spend a little more time on the details.

What is a cataract?

The human eye has a compound focusing system similar to that found in a camera. This system consists of the cornea, or curved clear window of the eye, an iris diaphragm to control the light entering the eye, and a crystalline or transparent lens located just behind the iris. A cataract is a clouding of the normally clear and transparent lens of the eye. It is not a tumor or a new growth of skin or tissue over the eye, but a fogging of the lens itself. When a cataract develops, the lens becomes cloudy like a frosted window and may cause a painless blurring of vision.

The lens, located behind the pupil, focuses light on the retina at the back of the eye to produce a sharp image. When a cataract forms, the lens can become so opaque and unclear that light cannot easily be transmitted to the retina. Often, however, a cataract covers only a small part of the lens and if sight is not greatly impaired, there is no need to remove the cataract. If a large portion of the lens becomes cloudy, sight can be partially or completely lost until the cataract is removed. When this blurring of vision becomes severe enough to interfere with the individual's daily activities, then cataract surgery may be necessary to restore visual function.

There are many misconceptions about cataracts. For instance, cataracts do not spread from eye to eye, though they may develop in both eyes at the same time. A cataract is not a film visible on the outside of the eye. Nor is it caused from overuse of the eyes or made worse by use of the eye. Cataracts rarely develop in a matter of months. They usually develop gradually over many years. Finally, cataracts are not related to cancer. Nor does having a cataract mean a person will be permanently blind. I told you there was some good news!

What causes cataracts to form?

Various conditions may cause cataracts to form: heredity is the determining factor in congenital and juvenile cataracts; toxic substances, certain eye injuries, chronic systemic disease (such as diabetes), or other specific eye diseases may cause cataracts. But, by far, the most common cause is simply the aging process. As we grow older, the lens gradually loses its water content and increases in density. The lens becomes hard in its center, and the ability to focus on near objects is diminished (usually requiring bifocals by age 45). As the lens ages it also becomes less clear.

These natural processes may set the stage for cataract formation. By age 60, according to some estimates, nearly two-thirds of the population develop the beginnings of cataracts. Cataracts usually develop bilaterally — in both eyes — but progress at different rates, so vision in one eye is often significantly better than the other.

Some degree of cataract formation is expected in virtually everyone over age 70. The time required for development of the cataract is anywhere from a few months to many years. The cataract may stop at an early stage of development and vision will then not be significantly affected. In other cases, the cataract continues to develop and interferes with vision.

Children as well as adults can develop cataracts. When cataracts appear in children, they are sometimes inherited. Or, they can be caused by an infection or inflammation during pregnancy that affects the unborn baby. This latter type of cataract is called congenital, meaning present at birth.

Eye injuries can cause cataracts in people of any age. A hard blow, puncture, cut, intense heat, or chemical burn can damage the lens and result in what is called a traumatic cataract. Certain infections, drugs, or diseases, such as diabetes, can also cause the lens to cloud and form a secondary cataract.

Does ultraviolet light cause cataracts

Researchers have claimed a causative relationship between exposure to UV (ultraviolet radiation) and cataracts. This claim is unjustified as the relationship is not proven and is highly unlikely. Dr. John Harding of England is an expert on cataracts and has written an excellent book on the subject and, as one reviewer of the book said: "He takes us through the epidemiological evidence purporting to show a role for sunlight in the development of cataracts and finds it wanting." One obvious point usually overlooked by the hand wringers, quaking and quivering before the evil sun god: *sunlight-related diseases do not correlate with the occurrence of cataracts.*

A more likely cause of cataracts is found at the other end of the light spectrum in the infrared range. Although ophthalmologists are generally smarter than the average doctor (you *have* to be just to spell ophth....), they suffer from the same semi-scientific mind set (cerebrus cementicus) as other scientists: if it's beyond their conception, and contrary to their training, then it can't exist or, if it does exist, it's wrong. So ophthalmologists push the UV causation of cataract formation without the slightest scientific evidence.

Dr. John Ott, the great pioneer in full-spectrum light and its importance to human health tried to penetrate this fire wall of prejudice, but was seldom successful. A classic example was when he applied to the American Cancer Society for a small grant for light research on cancer. The response was a classic example of cerebrus cementicus:

"The advisory committee has recommended disapproval of this application." The reason for this denial was that "results will be difficult to interpret in any meaningful way (and) no evidence exists or is presented to warrant the belief that such (effective light treatment) exists."

If that isn't defeatist enough, how about this don't-confuse-me-with-the-facts conclusion: "While there is every likelihood that exposure to different kinds of light will affect certain physiological responses in animals, they will only confuse the issue."

As a matter of fact, the UV phobics are looking at the wrong end of the light spectrum for the cause of cataracts. We know that the red end of the light spectrum, and especially the infrared portion (invisible like ultraviolet at the other end), is cataractogenic. One only has to examine glass blowers from the old school who had no eye protection. They continually looked into a special furnace that emitted primarily infrared light, not UV light. If they stuck to their profession, they all got "glass blowers cataract."

What is *your* consistent exposure to this cataract-forming infrared light? *Your ordinary, every day, incandescent light bulbs.*

What is your exposure to harmful ultraviolet rays? *NONE* as the atmosphere filters it out quite efficiently. (And don't worry about the "ozone hole"; that's more trash science.)

Detection and diagnosis

Usually cataracts cannot be viewed from the outside of the eye without proper instruments. If blurred vision or other symptoms are noticed, an ophthalmologist should be visited as soon as possible for a comprehensive medical eye examination.

The ophthalmologist examines the eye to determine the type, size, and location of the cataract. The interior of the eye is also viewed with an ophthalmoscope to determine if there are any other eye disorders contributing to the blurred vision.

Can cataracts be prevented or cured?

Although a large amount of research is currently underway, no preventive measures are known for cataracts that develop with the aging process. No diets, drugs, or medicines have been proven to delay or cure the developing cataract. (There are some things you can try, which we'll discuss at the end of this chapter.) But a safe surgical procedure, coupled with the appropriate corrective lenses, has preserved or restored sight for millions.

Treatment

When cataracts cause enough loss of sight to interfere with a person's work, hobbies, or lifestyle, it is time to remove them. Depending on individual needs, the patient and the ophthalmologist decide together when removal is necessary.

Surgery, which can be performed under general or local anesthesia, and often on an out-patient basis, is the only effective way to remove the cloudy lens from the eye.

Under ordinary circumstances, cataract surgery is not an emergency situation. There are only a few, rare instances where immediate action is indicated. Examples of these emergencies might be if the cataract causes glaucoma or if the eye is severely inflamed. Otherwise, the choice of whether or not to have surgery is up to the patient. If he or she decides to have the operation, the choice of when to have it is also his or hers to make.

In the past, surgeons usually waited until the cataract reached a mature or "ripe" stage to remove it. However, modern surgical advances have made it possible to perform this operation at any stage; usually as soon as the clouded lens begins to interfere significantly with comfort and normal daily activities.

But a word of caution: *Beware of the cataract cowboys.* These are the unscrupulous ophthalmologists who remove perfectly normal lenses for fun and profit. Their rationale, if they bother to have any at all, is that everyone eventually has to have cataract surgery so why not do it? It's hard to imagine why someone would go through the rigorous training, which demands a high degree of intelligence and a specialty that is regarded as highly as any in medicine, and then turn into a charlatan; but it is a fact of life. You could say the same thing about some preachers.

Cataracts cannot be removed with a laser. Ophthalmologic laser surgery can, however, be used later to open part of the lens membrane (capsule) if it becomes cloudy after cataract surgery. Rapidly changing technology and ongoing research has improved the treatment of cataracts in recent years. Eye drops, ointments, pills, special diets, or eye exercises have not been proven to dissolve or reduce a cataract. That doesn't mean you don't try everything you can before submitting to surgery. But, unfortunately, if you have cataracts and they are interfering with your vision, you will probably have to go through the operation.

Out of more than one million people who have cataracts removed each year in this country, over 95 percent obtain significant improvement in their vision. It is generally felt that it takes 20/40 (85 percent) or better vision to read average print. Thus we use 20/40 or better as a guide to successful surgery.

Will I have to wear glasses after cataract surgery?

Since cataract surgery removes the crystalline lens from the eye, a substitute lens must be provided if you are to be able to focus images onto your retina to enable you to see clearly.

Prior to the mid 1960s, nearly everyone wore thick cataract glasses to improve their vision following cataract surgery. The glasses were safe, simple, and relatively inexpensive. However, using them required some adjustment, for they magnified everything you saw by about 30 percent. This made things appear closer than they really were. These glasses also interfered with side vision and gave the wearer a tunnel-vision effect; so, to look from side to side, you had to turn your head. And for that person who had surgery on only one eye, the use of cataract glasses for one eye and regular glasses for the other created double vision because of the magnification problem.

Contact lenses eliminated some of the optical problems associated with cataract eye glasses. They did not significantly magnify image size and they provided good peripheral (side) vision. However, the greatest obstacle to the use of contact lenses was learning to successfully remove and insert the tiny lenses. Older people, particularly those with arthritis or tremors in the hands, found this task especially difficult. Even with the newer "extended wear" contact lenses for cataract patients, and the lenses created problems with eye irritation and/or infection. And if the patient has the dry eye problem mentioned earlier, obviously contact lenses are not practical.

Technological advances have greatly increased the ease of cataract success. The intraocular lens implant (IOL) offers significant advantages over cataract glasses and contact lenses, and lOLs are now the preferred method of visual rehabilitation for cataract patients. In fact, since the mid 1980s, lOLs have been implanted in virtually all cataract surgery patients. The IOL was truly one of the great medical achievements of the 20th century.

lOLs are made of space age plastics, which are well tolerated by the eye. Each IOL is specifically tailored to the individual visual needs of each patient.

The IOL is placed inside the eye at the end of a routine cataract extraction. It is placed in essentially the same location as the natural lens (cataract) that was removed, and it remains there permanently to provide the highest quality vision after cataract surgery.

Because the intraocular lens implant stays inside the eye, it never has to be handled, adjusted, or cleaned. Patients are free from having to depend on cumbersome external visual aids such as contact lenses or cataract glasses. Instead, most implant patients wear ordinary glasses or bifocals much the same as they did before their surgery. With the most recent advances in cataract and lens implant surgery, some people can even go without glasses.

More recently, the majority of cataracts have been removed by using a more modern technique known as extracapsular cataract extraction (ECCE). This technique permits the surgeon to suck out the cloudy contents within the lens capsule, but the thin capsule itself is left intact.

With this technique, a small space remains behind the pupil, and this makes it possible for the cataract surgeon to implant the plastic lens in the same place as the natural, cloudy lens that was removed. This maintains the natural anatomy of the eye and reduces the chances of complications associated with older methods. In addition, the extracapsular technique permits a smaller incision (10 mm), fewer or no sutures, and a shorter recovery period.

Phacoemulsification

Phacoemulsification (PE) is a newer form of extracapsular cataract extraction that permits the surgeon to remove the cloudy lens material through an even smaller incision (2-3 mm). Through this tiny incision, the surgeon, using the high magnification of an operating microscope, inserts a tiny hollow probe into the eye. The tip of this probe vibrates at ultrasonic speed to break up (emulsify) the lens. Then, by means of gentle suction, (aspiration) the lens fragments are removed, leaving the capsule intact. Often mistakenly called the "laser technique," phacoemulsification is the most sophisticated technique available for cataract surgery.

Phacoemulsification permits the smallest possible cataract incision, the fewest number of sutures, and the shortest recovery period. In the hands of an experienced cataract surgeon, phacoemulsification also reduces the incidence of complications and produces the best possible visual results.

What is no-stitch (sutureless) cataract surgery?

No-Stitch (sutureless) cataract surgery is the most recent advance in cataract surgery. Sutureless surgery is made possible by a revolutionary new way of constructing the small phacoemulsification incision. This new type of incision is self-sealing and requires no sutures. Yet it is even stronger and heals faster than earlier types of incisions, and with even fewer complications. With no-stitch surgery, cataract surgery patients are usually able to resume all normal activities within 24 hours after surgery. No-stitch or small incision surgery, combined with the latest small incision intraocular lenses, offers the cataract patient the best possible vision in the shortest possible time.

After cataract surgery, you may return almost immediately to all but the most strenuous activities. You will have to take eye drops as your ophthalmologist directs. Several postoperative visits are needed to check on the progress of the eye as it heals.

Note: It is important to understand that complications during or after surgery can occur. With any surgical procedure, no matter how sophisticated and successful, the possibility of complications always exists. Fortunately, with modern cataract surgery, complications are relatively rare and when they do occur, the condition can usually be corrected. However, unexpected serious complications can occur and they can cause a permanent decrease in vision. It is therefore necessary that you be fully informed as to the risks and benefits of your contemplated surgery.

And one further caveat: Choose your cataract surgeon carefully. If you have a cataract problem, I strongly suggest that you contact the American Society of Cataract and Refractive Surgery for a referral in your area. Their number is 800-451-1339.'

Before submitting to surgery

As I said earlier, if you have cataracts that are inhibiting your ability to see, you'll probably have to go through with sur-

33

gery. But before your cataracts get that far along, I suggest you try a few things at home that may prevent the cataract from getting worse and may even help some.

The most important fighters of cataracts are antioxidants, including vitamins A, C, and E. These are absolutely vital! I've preached these for so long that I'm sure you think I'm a broken record. But don't take this recommendation lightly. Vitamin C alone has demonstrated the ability to halt the progression of cataracts.

If you have a cataract forming, I suggest you take as much as 25,000 IU of vitamin A (unless you're pregnant); 1,000 mg of vitamin C, three times a day; and 800-1,200 IU of vitamin E.

In addition to these antioxidants, I heartily recommend you take either Pycnogenol or Healthy Resolve's Herbal Antioxidants, especially if you're a diabetic. These antioxidants, coupled with those mentioned above, can reverse early cataracts and halt more developed ones.

Many alternative doctors and researchers also believe that it's important to take at least 200 meg of selenium in order to prevent or halt the development of cataracts. Researchers have found that many cataract sufferers are selenium deficient. This doesn't prove cause and effect, but I wouldn't take any chances. You probably need the extra selenium anyway.

Herbal remedies

If your desire is to use herbal remedies, I've got a few interesting ones that many people swear by — including my great-grandmother Lucy Bell.

The first is relatively simple. It's called celery juice. All you have to do is smash some freshly picked celery into a pulp with a fork, add equal parts water, and apply the juice to your eyes a few times a week with a dropper. After it begins to work, you can reduce the frequency to a few times a month.

An even easier remedy is coconut milk. With a dropper, apply the milk to the eye and lay down for 10 minutes with hot damp cloths over your eyes. If you catch your cataract early enough, only one treatment will be necessary. Of course, I don't think it would hurt to do it two or three times over the course of a month.

Other herbs that you might want to try in an eye wash are chervil and eyebright (see page 37 for the recipe) or the entire snap dragon plant. The best recipe I've seen for the snap dragon plant was in John Heinerman's *Encyclopedia of Fruits, Vegetables, and Herbs* (Parker, 1988). His recipe: "Bring one quart of distilled water (very important to use only this kind) to a rolling boil. Add one heaping handful of carefully cleaned and coarsely chopped fresh root. Cover with a tight-fitting lid, reduce heat and simmer 15 minutes exactly. Remove promptly from the heat, uncover, and add the cut and chopped contents of one small-to-medium snap dragon. Cover again and steep for an hour. Strain twice, bottle, and refrigerate. Makes the best eye wash you've ever seen. Bathe eyes frequently with an eye cup as needed."

Heinerman also says that aloe vera gel rubbed over the closed eyelid (but not in the eye!) will also help cataracts in the early stages.

Retinal Detachment

Imagine that your eye is like a camera, and the retina is the film. The retina is a fine sheet of nerve tissue lining the inside of the eye. Rays of light enter the eye and are focused on the retina by the lens. The retina produces a picture, which is sent along the optic nerve for the brain to interpret. It's rather like the film in the camera being developed, but in this case it's being developed continuously!

The retina is attached to the inner surface of the eye. If there is a tear or hole in the retina then fluid can get underneath it. This weakens the attachment so that the retina becomes detached — rather like wallpaper peeling off a damp wall.

When this happens, the retina cannot compose a clear picture from the incoming rays and your vision becomes blurred and dim.

Detachment of the retina happens more to middle-aged, short-sighted people. It is uncommon however and only about one person in 10,000 is affected. Very rarely, younger people can have a weakness of the retina, or it can detach as a result of a blow to the head.

The most common symptom is a shadow spreading across the vision of one eye. If you get help early, it may be necessary to have only a laser or freezing treatment. This is usually performed under a local anesthetic. Often however, an operation to repair the hole in the retina will be needed. This is usually done under a general anesthetic and can be repaired with a single operation in 90 percent of the cases. This does not usually cause much pain, but your eye will be sore and swollen for a few days afterward. You will usually need to stay in the hospital for two or three days after your operation.

How much vision can you expect after a successful operation? This depends on how much the retina has detached and for how long. The shadow caused by the detachment will disappear in all cases when the retina has been put back in place. However, if the detachment involves the part of the retina that's responsible for your central vision, the macula, this may not recover. The longer this part of the retina has been detached, the smaller the chance that your central vision will recover to its former level. But, if this is the case, you will still have some useful vision left.

What happens if the retina is not put back in place? Most people will lose all useful vision if no operation is carried out, or if the treatment is unsuccessful. Occasionally, if the detachment involves the lower portion of the retina, some vision may recover by itself.

Generally, you can't prevent retinal attachment. It doesn't happen as a result of straining your eyes, bending, or heavy lifting. If your family has a history of retinal detachment, or your doctor finds a weakness in your retina, then preventive laser or freezing treatment may be needed. In most cases, however, it's not possible to take preventive action.

If you have had a retinal detachment in one eye you are at increased risk of developing one in the other eye. But there is only about a one in ten chance of this happening.

What if your sight cannot be fully restored? Much can be done to help you use your remaining vision as fully as possible. You should ask your doctor to refer you to the a "low-vision" specialist. There are a variety of optical aids such as brighter reading lights, simple magnifying glasses, and more sophisticated equipment that can help you.

One herbal eyewash that I've found to be especially helpful for retinal detachment is made from chervil and other herbs. The formula is from France and was created by Professor Leon Binet, a former dean of the Faculty of Medicine in Paris. "His remedy calls for equal parts (or one tablespoon each) of freshly cut chervil, parsley, Roman chamomile (*Anthemis nobilis*, not German chamomile), and lavender flowers, all to be added to one pint of boiling water and permitted to steep away from any heat for about 20-30 minutes. I recommend that an equal amount (one tbsp) of fresh or dried eyebright herb also be added to the solution, which is later strained and applied to both eyes with an eye cup three times a day. This is good for cataracts, detached retinas, and occasionally glaucoma." (*Heinerman's Encyclopedia of Fruits, Vegetables, and Herbs*, Parker, 1988)

Diabetic Retinopathy

About one person in 50 in the U.S. is affected by diabetes mellitus, or "sugar diabetes." This means that the body cannot cope normally with sugar and other carbohydrates in the diet.

People with diabetes face a risk of eye disease that can cost them their sight if they don't get regular eye exams. The disease is called diabetic retinopathy, and it's a leading cause of blindness and visual impairment in the U.S.

Although it's not clear whether diabetic retinopathy can be prevented, it can be slowed — and vision preserved — by laser or other surgical treatment. For best results, treatment must be given at particular times during the course of the disease. For that reason, regular medical attention is important.

Most sight loss from diabetic retinopathy can be prevented. But it is vital that it be diagnosed early. You may not realize there is anything wrong with your eyesight, so regular eye checks are extremely important.

Blood vessel damage

Retinopathy results from damage to microscopic blood vessels in the retina, the light-sensing membrane in the back of the eye. Diabetes damages blood vessels in the eye, just as it does those in the heart, kidneys and other areas of the body, although researchers aren't sure how.

In retinopathy, blood vessel linings weaken, sometimes bulging out to form tiny aneurysms — sac-like dilations in the vessel wall. The micro aneurysms and vessels then begin to leak fluid into the retina, causing it to thicken.

At this early stage, called background retinopathy, sight may not be affected. But if the retinal swelling (edema) affects the center of the macula (the central part of the retina that's responsible for detailed vision), reading and other close work may become difficult.

As diabetes damages the blood vessels, they may leak fluids, fats, protein, and blood. Not infrequently, such leakage creates fluid accumulations in the macular region. This causes swelling of the retina and blurred or impaired vision.

The blood vessel changes that occur in retinopathy aren't visible without special instruments. And because the retina has no pain receptors, retinopathy isn't painful.

The disease begins and may progress without warning until a person notices a blurring or even a total block in vision. That's why regular eye exams are so important for diabetics.

The longer a person has diabetes, the more likely he will develop retinopathy. About half of those who have been insulin-dependent for 14 years have some vascular damage in the retina. Thus, retinopathy is more common in people with juvenile-onset diabetes than in those with adult-onset diabetes. Nonetheless, it's just as important for people with adult-onset disease to have regular eye exams because their diabetes may have begun several years before it was diagnosed.

Sight-saving treatments

"Background retinopathy" that isn't affecting sight isn't treatable. But the disease will need to be watched closely.

Close monitoring allows vision-threatening changes, such as macular edema and proliferative retinopathy, to be detected and treated immediately to prevent irreversible vision loss. Surgical treatments can prevent deterioration of vision in 60 percent of patients.

Laser surgery is the standard procedure used to stop or reverse damaging changes in blood vessels. The treatment works by sealing off, or photocoagulating, bleeding vessels.

The laser also can be used to stop abnormal blood vessel growth. In a technique called "scatter photocoagulation," several small burns are made around the perimeter of the retina, where they have little effect on vision. By reducing the amount of retinal tissue that uses oxygen, the treatment allows the more important, central part of the retina to receive the oxygen it needs. Therefore, new blood vessels with the potential to cause problems are less likely to form there. Laser surgery usually is performed by subspecialists in retinal surgery, who can do the procedure in their offices.

In severe cases of retinopathy, a surgical procedure called vitrectomy can improve sight. Vitrectomy removes blood that has leaked into the vitreous. The procedure improves vision in many people, but not without some risk. Various complications occur in 25 percent of the procedures. Vitrectomy is performed in a hospital operating room, often on an outpatient basis.

Physicians don't yet know whether patients can do anything to prevent retinopathy or keep it from getting worse. Evidence suggests that controlling blood sugar might be the key. As yet, however, the success of this strategy hasn't been proven.

The best a patient can do is to try to control blood sugar as well as possible. That includes dieting, watching sugar intake and monitoring blood sugar levels.

Macular Degeneration

Over the years, I've received a lot of mail asking about possible natural cures for macular degeneration (MD). Unfortunately, there hasn't been a lot of cures to talk about. But there are plenty of things that can keep this disease from progressing or starting in the first place. So you can understand what's happening with the treatments, a quick biology class is needed.

Simply stated, macular degeneration is damage or breakdown of the macula. As the eye looks straight ahead, the macula is the point of the retina where light rays meet as they are focused by the cornea and the lens of the eye. Similar to the film in a camera, the retina receives the images that come through the "camera-like" lens. If the macula is damaged, the central part of the images is blocked as if a blurred area had been placed in the center of the picture, but the images around the blurred area may be seen clearly.

The macula is very important and is responsible for what we see straight in front of us, the vision needed for detailed activities such as reading and writing and our ability to appreciate color.

The eye still sees objects to the side, since side or "peripheral" vision is usually not affected. For this reason, macular degeneration alone will not cause total blindness. Even people with the most severe form of the disease are capable of taking care of themselves. However, it can make reading or close work difficult or impossible without the use of special low-vision optical aids.

The retina is the delicate layer of tissue that lines the inside wall of the back of the eye. The macula is a very small area in the center of the retina. In size, the macula is about the same as a capital "O" in the type of this pamphlet.

Although macular degeneration most often occurs in older people, aging alone does not always result in central visual loss. Nevertheless, macular degeneration is the leading cause of impairment of reading and fine "close-up" vision in the United States.

Causes and symptoms

The most common form of macular degeneration is called dry macular degeneration. This form accounts for 70 percent of all cases, and is associated with aging. It is, by far, the leading cause of impaired vision in the over-65 population. It is caused by a breakdown or thinning of the tissues in the macula.

About 10 percent of macular degeneration falls into a category called wet or exudative macular degeneration. Normally, the macula is protected by a thin tissue that separates it from very fine blood vessels nourishing the back of the eye. Sometimes these blood vessels break or leak and cause scar tissue to form. This often leads to the growth of new abnormal blood vessels in the scar tissue. These newly formed vessels are especially fragile. They rupture easily and may leak. Blood and leaking fluid destroy the macula and cause further scarring. Vision becomes distorted and blurred and dense scar tissue blocks out central vision to a severe degree.

Other types of macular degeneration are inherited. It may occur in juveniles (juvenile macular degeneration) or occasionally, injury, infection, or inflammation may damage the delicate tissue of the macula.

Macular degeneration can cause different symptoms in different people. Sometimes only one eye loses vision while the other eye continues to see well for many years. If only one eye is affected, macular degeneration is hardly noticeable in the beginning stages, particularly when the other eye is completely normal. This condition often involves one eye at a time, so it may be some time before a patient notices visual problems.

Color vision may become dim and other visual symptoms can develop due to macular degeneration: Words on a page look blurred; straight lines look distorted and, in some cases, the center of vision looks more distorted than the rest of the scene; A dark or empty area appears in the center of vision.

Many patients do not realize they have a macular problem until blurred vision becomes obvious. Your ophthalmologist can detect macular degeneration in the early stages by viewing the macula with an instrument called an ophthalmoscope.

Macular degeneration can be detected and diagnosed early. Early detection is important since people may not realize their vision is impaired. Having your eyes checked is especially appropriate if other family members have a history of retinal problems. For patients with macular degeneration, early diagnosis by an ophthalmologist may prevent further damage and aid the individual in making a visual adjustment with low-vision aids.

Surgical treatment

There is no cure for the most common dry forms of macular degeneration. However, ophthalmologic laser surgery has been used to retard the spread of the less common wet (exudative) form, but only if this treatment is applied in the very early stages of the condition. In this treatment, a focused intense beam of laser light is used to seal off leaking membranes and destroy new blood vessels. This reduces further loss of vision from progressive scarring of the macula and the surrounding retina. It is obviously a destructive technique, like back-burning to stop a forest fire, but sometimes necessary.

Drug therapy

Most everyone remembers thalidomide, the tranquilizer that caused grotesque deformities in babies. But if you are not pregnant the drug has some remarkable therapeutic properties. It is excellent in the treatment of leprosy and the use of this drug is partially responsible for the discontinuance of the inhumane leper colonies that debased the lives of millions over the centuries.

Another remarkable property of this drug is its ability to stop the growth of blood vessels in the retina that cause a displacement of the retina in wet macular degeneration. The thalidomide acts as an "angiogenesis inhibitor," an inhibitor of blood-vessel growth.

But many patients, such as Woodrow Wirsig who reported his dilemma in the *Wall Street Journal*, are being denied treatment. In Wirsig's case, the FDA says he's too blind in one eye and not blind enough in the other to qualify for treatment!

The 1962 Keefauver bill, which put the FDA into the practice of medicine, must be repealed. Ask your congressman if he supports legislation to eliminate the effectiveness section of the 1962 bill. Determining if a particular drug or device is effective is the place of the doctor and his patient, not ignorant and venal bureaucrats.

Just how bad is the FDA for your health? According to one qualified critic of the FDA, Dr. Robert Goldberg, although 82 percent of bio-tech drugs are created in this country, 75 percent are used in Europe and not the U.S. Some of the drugs eventually are used here, but how many people like Mr. Wirsig will go partially blind in the interim? *(Wall Street Journal,* March 11, 1996; *Insider Report,* February 1996.)

Optical aids and lighting

Low-vision optical aids often improve vision for people with macular degeneration. Many different types of magnifying devices are available. Spectacles, hand or stand magnifiers, telescopes, and closed circuit television for viewing objects are some of the available resources. Aids are either prescribed by your ophthalmologist or by referral to a low-vision specialist or center. Bright illumination properly directed for reading and close work are often beneficial. Special lamps can also be helpful. Books, newspapers, and other items available in large print offer further help.

A patient who already has macular degeneration can be helped. Fortunately, visual aids are available to assist many patients in leading a comfortable and relatively normal life. With these devices and proper motivation, people with visual loss can often read, do modified close-up work, and continue to take care of themselves.

If you are over age 50, or if your family has a history or retinal problems, you should have your eyes checked periodically for signs of eye problems like macular degeneration. Early detection and subsequent treatment, if indicated, may help prevent additional visual loss.

Nutritional help

Can vitamins and minerals help to alleviate macular degeneration? Even the conservative American Academy of Ophthalmology (AAO) agrees, conditionally, that zinc can help. Zinc is highly concentrated in the eye, particularly in the retina and tissues surrounding the macula. Zinc is necessary for the action of over 100 enzymes, including chemical reactions in the retina. Studies have shown that some older people have low levels of zinc in their blood, either because of poor diet or poor absorption of zinc from food. Because zinc is important for the health of the macula, some doctors, including me, think that supplements of zinc in the diet may slow down macular degeneration.

And better still, the research supports our theory. In February 1996, researchers at the Department of Veteran Affairs announced the results of a study related to macular degeneration in the elderly. A study of U.S. veterans, published in *the Journal of the American Optometric Association*, found that taking a natural combination of nutrients, which includes zinc and vitamins C and E appeared to prevent the progression of age related macular degeneration.

This is great news and offers hope to thousands of older Americans with early symptoms of macular degeneration. Finally, there is scientific evidence that proves antioxidant therapy, led by zinc, can perhaps slow the progression of this leading cause of blindness. I suggest 25-100 mg of zinc picolinate daily (picolinate is more easily absorbed by the body).

A vitamin/mineral program may also help. Here's why: Chemical reactions from light in the eye activate oxygen that may cause macular damage. Logic dictates, then, that antioxidants may help to limit these unwanted chemical reactions that can lead to macular degeneration. The best known antioxidants are vitamins E, C, and A, along with selenium, zinc (of course), taurine (an amino acid), and beta-carotene (in spite of the recent negative press). The new herbal antioxidants are also important.

All of these nutrients are very important for the eye to function properly, especially zinc and taurine. Some people have been helped by the simply adding vitamin E and selenium supplements. And still others have had zinc and selenium administered intravenously before their eyesight improved.

Researchers at the University of Illinois found that failing to get enough vitamin A in your diet makes you twice as likely to develop macular degeneration. If you are noticing MD symptoms, bump your intake of vitamin A up to 25,000 IU.

Again, the research about zinc and other supplements in the treatment of macular degeneration is still ongoing. My evidence shows that it's more likely that zinc does indeed help to fight macular degeneration. My advice is to take your zinc and other antioxidants. Complete dosages for these nutrients are on page 61.

A hormonal treatment

In their book *The Melatonin Miracle* (Simon & Schuster, 1995), Drs. Pierpaoli and Regelson indicate that melatonin may be an important ingredient in the treatment of macular degeneration. They write:

"We have firsthand knowledge of one case in which melatonin completely reversed ... macular degeneration.... At our suggestion, several years ago our friend began taking melatonin. After a few weeks, he reported that he had begun to notice a gradual change for the better in his vision. Within a few months, he said that his vision had returned. Wondering whether he was experiencing some kind of placebo effect, we declined to take his word for it. His ophthalmologist and later other doctors verified our friend's claim, confirming that he had indeed been cured and that this was the first time they had ever seen macular degeneration heal itself. Although the doctors did not quite believe that melatonin was the reason, they conceded they could offer no other rational explanation.... Based on this event, clinical trials are now planned to determine whether melatonin could be an effective treatment for macular degeneration."

The doctors went on to explain that melatonin normalizes zinc levels, so if you decide to try melatonin, make sure you're also taking all of the vitamins and minerals mentioned above.

As I've said before, melatonin is a "miracle hormone" if there ever was one. As with most medical treatments, it won't work in every instance, but you might want to give it a try. Melatonin supplements usually come in three mg tablets. But if you're in your early 40s, that's three times as much as you need (one mg). If you fall into the 45-54 age group, I recommend taking half a tablet (1.5 mg) before you go to bed at night. If you are between 55 and 65, you can take a full tablet, if half doesn't do the trick. And folks over 65 can take as much as two tablets. You can order melatonin from Healthy Resolve at 800-728-2288.

Herbal treatments

There are two herbs that you should also use to treat this disease. The first is bilberry, which we discuss in full detail on page 63.

46

The other herb is called Ginkgo biloba. Many elderly patients who suffer from senile macular degeneration have found that Ginkgo biloba extracts have helped tremendously. Currently, there is more evidence supporting the use of bilberry, so I recommend you use it first. If you decide to try Ginkgo biloba, (20 mgs, twice a day, of the 24 percent ginkgo flavonglycoside extract), you should be able to find it at your health food store.

And finally, one of my own favorites: milk thistle. I have yet to find a lot of supporting data on how this one works with macular degeneration, but it's such a good antioxidant that it can't hurt to try. I think it should be a part of your daily supplement regimen whether you suffer from MD or not. Take 10-100 mgs of milk thistle.

With all of these treatment options, one clear fact is that the sooner MD is diagnosed, the more likely a treatment plan may work to save the vision. This is yet another reason for people in their 60s and older to have regular, yearly examinations by an optometrist or ophthalmologist.

Glaucoma: Stealing Your Sight

Although it is a relatively rare condition, glaucoma — a leading cause of blindness in the United States — receives a lot of attention in the media. This is because most of the cases of blindness due to glaucoma are thought to be preventable. I've always thought there were alternative treatments that might be effective, but until recently, most people just weren't receptive to alternatives.

While we don't have any conclusive evidence of any treatment to cure glaucoma, I have made a few minor remarks about its treatment through the years. But my interest was peaked by a letter from a subscriber who said, "Do you know that cannabis, marijuana, has been prescribed for years for glaucoma?" I had known this, but didn't know how widespread the knowledge was.

Then during the 1996 elections, several Western states passed laws allowing doctor's to prescribe marijuana and other "illegal" drugs for medical purposes. While these new laws indicate a revolution in health care — people are finally taking charge of their own health — you can be sure Big Brother will squash them like an ant. So much for self government.

Anyway, this report won't deal with marijuana as a therapy (because you already know about it — and I don't want to get raided by the FDA, ATF, and FBI). But I would like to say that I think you should be allowed to use whatever medical treatments you need to help your body heal. I can list too many instances where the government thought they were helping when, in fact, they were doing more harm. (And please don't try to order this therapy from the folks at Healthy Resolve — they won't be able to help you with this one.)

I mentioned that glaucoma is one of the leading causes of blindness, but there is some good news: It can be prevented if you begin treatment soon enough. Unfortunately, the early signs of glaucoma are difficult to detect, and all too often people don't notice the early symptoms, they wait too long before they seek treatment, and blindness is the sad result.

Glaucoma causes disease of the optic nerve. When pressure inside the eye begins to increase, damage to the optic nerve can be the result. If this includes damage to the nerve fibers, blind spots can develop.

Studies of many thousands of patients find that most people have an eye pressure less than 20 units of pressure in each eye without optic nerve damage. (You can have glaucoma with less pressure; you might not have glaucoma even if your pressure is higher. The "20 units" rule relates to most, but not all patients.)

There are various types of glaucoma (30 in all), including chronic open-angle glaucoma and angle-closure glaucoma. The former is the most prevalent, accounting for 90 percent of all adult glaucoma. Chronic open-angle is the insidious kind of glaucoma — often taking your sight before you realize there has been any damage.

With angle-closure glaucoma, the drainpipe becomes completely blocked. The symptoms are recognizable and can include blurred vision, severe eye pain, headaches, rainbow haloes around lights, and nausea and vomiting. If you experience any of these symptoms, get help immediately.

Note: If you are of Asian or African ancestry, your risk of angular-closure glaucoma is higher than the general population.

One probable cause of glaucoma that you might not have thought about is your pharmaceutical drugs. The *Physicians Desk Reference* list 94 medications that can cause glaucoma, including steroids, oral contraceptives, gold, and antihistamines. Ask your doctor if your medication has glaucoma as one of its side effects. You may even want to go to the library and check out all the side effects of your medication in the *Physicians Desk Reference* — your doctor may not know.

Detection and Treatment

During a complete eye exam, your doctor will perform a series of tests, which can include a measurement of your intraocular pressure, a look at how well your eye is draining, an evaluation of any optic nerve damage, and a test of your visual field.

Whether you receive any or all of these tests depends upon your risk factors. These factors include your age, ancestry, nearsightedness, eye injuries, and a family history of glaucoma.

As a rule, damage caused by glaucoma cannot be reversed. Eye drops, medications, and laser and surgical operations are used to prevent or slow further damage from occurring.

Glaucoma is usually controlled with eye drops taken several times a day, sometimes in combination with medications by mouth. These medications decrease eye pressure, either by slowing the production of aqueous fluid within the eye or by improving the flow leaving the drainage angle.

You should notify your ophthalmologist immediately if you think you may be experiencing any of the following side effects: a stinging sensation, red eyes, blurred vision, head-aches, or changes in pulse, heartbeat, or breathing.

The drugs used to treat glaucoma can cause (among other things): tingling of fingers and toes, drowsiness, loss of appetite, anemia, and taste disturbances .

If you use eye drops for glaucoma, you need to be particularly wary of other medications. The *Annals of Internal Medicine* (112,2:120) reports that these prescription eye drops can react with other medications after being absorbed into the body through tear ducts. (The eye drops can also cancel out the benefits of some medications, such as diabetes and asthma drugs.)

The side effects from these reactions can cause headache, disorientation, tremors, and lower heart rate and blood pressure. If you have any of these symptoms, see your doctor immediately.

There is a way you can avoid most of these complications. Simply lie down while applying the drops (one at a time) and, using a Kleenex, apply light pressure to the inside corner of your eye for four or five minutes. This will block the tear ducts and let the medicine do its job on the eye.

Laser surgery

Laser surgery treatments may be effective for different types of glaucoma. The laser is usually used in one of two ways. In open-angle glaucoma, the drain itself is treated. The laser is used to enlarge the drain (trabeculoplasty) to help control eye pressure. In angle-closure glaucoma, the laser creates a hole in the iris (iridotomy) to improve the flow of aqueous fluid to the drain.

Laser treatment is only necessary in a small percentage of cases (10 percent or so) — patients who simply do not respond to traditional glaucoma treatments. According to Dr. Paul N. Schacknow, an ophthalmologist who performs laser surgery, the laser usually works to lower eye pressure in about 80 percent of patients for whom it is appropriate. "While for unknown reasons, it doesn't work in about 20 percent of open-angle glaucoma patients, it doesn't appear to harm them in any way either."

These are the conventional methods of treatment you're sure to hear when you go to the eye doctor for treatment of glaucoma. Generally, these methods will work to keep glaucoma from progressing. But there are also some natural remedies that can be tried before resorting to the above procedures (if you're early in the disease's progression) or in conjunction with them.

Nutritional therapy

There are several things you can do at home to reduce the pressure involved in glaucoma. The first step is to make sure you're taking all the nutrients mentioned at the end of this report. In many cases, these are the minimum amount of nutrients that your eye needs. With glaucoma, you'll need to boost several of these to much greater levels. We'll discuss this in a moment.

First, you need to find out if the higher pressure in your eye is being caused by allergies. Avoiding known allergens has been shown to lower the eye pressure by as much as 20 millimeters. This may not solve your problem entirely, but it's the best place to begin. Also, make sure you're avoiding sugar and processed foods.

Once you identified and avoided the things you're allergic to, it's time to add additional supplements to your diet.

Start by adding megadoses of vitamin C. Some doctors recommend taking 500 mg of C for every two kilograms (2.2 pounds) of body weight. I think this might be a little high. Start with around 20,000 mg and work your way up to this dosage. If you notice any problems, reduce the dosage to a comfortable level. With dosages this high, you'll probably want to work in conjunction with a holistic doctor. As the pressure goes down, see if you can reduce the dosage without allowing the pressure to go up again.

Other nutrients that I've discussed in the pages of my newsletters that are crucial for the treatment of glaucoma are bioflavonoids and magnesium. The bioflavonoids are so crucial to your health, including the health of your eye, that I told

Healthy Resolve to include them in their Maximum multivitamin. A healthy person needs only about 100 mgs a day, but for glaucoma sufferers, 1,000 mgs a day is more appropriate.

As for magnesium, a report in the journal *Ophthalmologica* indicates that 122 mg of magnesium daily can improve visual field defects by increasing the blood flow to the eye. I suggest you take as much magnesium as your body can handle. Start with 500 mg and work your way up. If you begin to experience diarrhea, cut back until it goes away.

Herbal healing

In his book *Encyclopedia of Fruits, Vegetables, and Herbs,* John Heinerman discusses the wisdom of Maria Treben, a renowned German folk healer and popular herbalist. Heinerman says, "Maria Treben insists that glaucoma is not an eye disorder, but rather a definite malfunction of the kidneys instead. A tea should be made, she observes, from equal parts of stinging nettle, yarrow, calendula, and horsetail, and 2-3 cups consumed each day. Bring 1 qt. of water to a boil, add these herbs, cover and simmer for seven minutes; then remove and steep another 45 minutes. Strain and sweeten with honey before drinking."

I don't know if this concoction will work or not, as I've never tried it on any of my patients. But if you have glaucoma, it couldn't hurt to try it. If it works, let me know. I have to admit that I'm a little suspicious, though. The Chinese say the liver is connected to the eyes, not the kidneys. But if a remedy works, who am I to argue,

Heinerman, in his revised and expanded version of the aforementioned book (Reward, 1995), also tells of a glaucoma treatment that he got from an Egyptian pharmaceutical student. He says that "the finest sesame oil should be used."

Here's how: "First, about half a cup of the oil needs to be cooked until it is rather hot." The best way to heat the oil is to put it into an empty baby-food jar. Then place the jar into about two inches of boiling water and allow to heat. "When the oil is very hot to the touch, remove from the pan and strain through several layers of gauze. Allow to thoroughly cool until the oil is comfortably warm. This can be tested by simply dropping a little bit on the tip of the tongue. The, using an eyedropper, put three drops of this oil into each eye just before retiring for the night."

Hormonal therapy

If none of the above treatments works to slow, halt, or reverse your glaucoma, would you be willing to try something a little unusual? Of course you would. Unfortunately, you'll have to do some research, because it's extremely difficult to find. But if you find it, you'll be amazed at how well it works in most cases, so read on.

You've probably never heard of Emanuel Josephson, M.D., but neither have most doctors. He was born in 1895, so he would be over 100 years old if alive today. But his great clinical work on glaucoma is still remembered by a few of us. I came across his name again when I was doing research on my monograph about hormone therapies. As I mentioned in that report, one of the great tragedies in medicine was the government's suppression of the use of adrenal cortical extract, or ACE. You can read in depth about ACE in my report, *Hormone Replacement Therapies* (to order, call Rhino Publishing 1-888-317-6767 or 416-352-5126).

The adrenal cortex, the outer layers of the adrenal glands which are located on top of your kidneys, is a treasure house of life-sustaining hormones. Among other duties, hormones of the adrenal cortex regulate your water balance and the electrolytes (minerals) essential to life. Dr. Josephson reasoned that since glaucoma was basically a problem of fluid control in the eye, too much in and too little out, a deficiency of the hormones of the adrenal cortex might be at least part of the problem. He proved to be right and, over his career, successfully treated many cases of glaucoma. In fact, he had a 72 *percent success rate* in early cases.

So adrenal deficiency and glaucoma go hand in hand but, even today — 50 years after Josephson's discovery —

few doctors make the diagnosis of adrenal deficiency. Even if they did recognize adrenal deficiency, they *still* wouldn't get the connection with glaucoma. Dr. Josephson remarked sadly: "My hope and expectation that ophthalmology would welcome (ACE) has been rudely shattered." To obtain ACE you will have to go to one of the medically-free countries such as Mexico.

If you do find a clinic that uses quality ACE and the treatment works for you, please write us and tell us all the details. We'd love to hear about it.

Eye Treatments You Can Do At Home

In the course of doing this report, I came across a large body of information concerning the value of massage as it relates to improving eyesight. I'm not an expert at this; I do understand the theory behind massage, and I suspect it coincides with Dr. William Bates' theories on relaxation discussed on page 10. What better way to relax that with a full-body massage?

Tension and strain cause numerous medical difficulties, including eyestrain and poor vision. Sight problems are almost always accompanied by patterns of muscle tension and weakness. For example, those who suffer with myopia tend to have pronounced tension in the forehead, jaw, neck, shoulders and upper arms, lower back, and often in the calves. With this in mind, here are some suggestions for various massage points that may help improve your vision naturally. The instructions below are for "self massage." I would expect better results from a professional Masseuse.

Begin with a body massage.

Notice which areas of the face are the most tense — we'll come back to these areas in a minute. Now do a neck massage and shoulder rotations. And, with the aid of someone, have the back massaged — and also your legs and calves if you have tension in these areas.

Now, massage your face

Warm your fingers by rubbing them together and begin with your jaw. Always begin very gently and spend a couple of minutes on each area. Work outward from the point of your chin under and behind the ears. The point directly under the ears is often very tight. Opening and closing the jaw is a good idea as well as yawning. Work from the bridge of the nose outward over the cheekbones and up toward the temples. Use circular strokes on the temples. Continue on the eyebrows, working outward from the center using long strokes. Use your fingertips to stretch out the brow, and alternate with picking up the brow with your thumb and forefinger and stretching it out. Often a point between the brow is very tense, use small circular motions on this area. Another delicate point is in the indentation outside the bridge of the nose on the inner edge of the eyebrows. Work above and below the brows and finally use long strokes on the forehead.

Notice how your face and your eyes feel. You will find you have your own pattern of tension that you can subsequently pay special attention to.

Massaging your neck

Turn your head to one side, feel along from behind the ear down to your chest and you will find the side neck flexor or sternocleidomastoid. This muscle can become tighter than any other muscle in the body. Some people have mistaken this muscle for a bone. Gently at first, until it warms up, palpate, tap, and stroke it. Do each side, then massage the back of the neck working out from the spine. The top of the spine at the very base of the skull is often quite tight. Finally, finish by doing head rotations. Start with small rotations, in each direction do a dozen circles gradually expanding to your full range of motion. Always do rotations slowly and deliberately.

Stretching the muscles of the eye

Close both eyes tightly, hold your lids shut firmly, squeezing. Then open them suddenly, arching your brows and stretching your face. Repeat several times.

Look up as far as possible, look down as far as possible, inhale on up, and exhale on down. Then blink rapidly a dozen or so times. Look as far right as possible, look as far left as possible and blink rapidly again. Look diagonally up to left, down to right, up to right, down to left, and blink rapidly. Attempt to look in back of yourself.

Full range of motion eye rotations. Rotate your eyes around the periphery of your vision. Always do these slowly and deliberately. Concentrate on one eye at a time, then try both. Go around a dozen or so times then go around the other direction the same number of times. Try rotations with your eyes shut.

How often should you stretch the muscles of the eye? Whenever you feel them to be tight or constricted or having a limited range of motion, at least several times a day. Some people find that after they have been wearing glasses or contacts and remove them the muscles of the eye are especial "sticky," and don't move freely.

The Eastern approach

As usual, the Chinese have a different philosophy. I came across some interesting data about various Chinese exercises, acupuncture, and herbs. I offer it here for your information, but make no claim to its efficacy. All I can say is there is more than one approach to health care.

And you can't argue with success: In China, students perform eye exercises twice a day, for about 10 minutes, as do factory workers. As a result, China seems to have a much lower rate of myopia than the U.S. (The Chinese do not spend hours watching TVs or computer monitors, either — but that too is changing.) So, if you're so inclined, try a bit of Chinese massage.

I do, however, recommend caution when it comes to various Chinese herbs. The quality of the Chinese herbs found in America is often questionable.

Acupressure

Acupressure is excellent for relieving eye strain and fatigue. If you find any of the listed pressure points to be sensitive, it's likely that you are indeed suffering from eyestrain.

To perform acupressure correctly, gradually apply pressure to each of the points, then hold the pressure without movement for three minutes. One minute of steady pressure calms and relaxes. To stimulate an area, apply pressure for only four to five seconds. The pressure should be somewhere between firm and outright pain. The more developed the muscles the more pressure can be applied.

The points

"Drilling Bamboo" (B2): In the indentations outside the bridge of the nose on the inner edge of the eyebrows.

"Four Whites" (St2): Half an inch below the center of the lower eye ridge in an indentation of the cheek.

"Facial Beauty" (St3): At the bottom of the cheek bone directly in line with the pupil of the eye.

"Heavenly Pillar" (BIO): Half an inch below the base of the skull on the ropy muscles, half an inch outward from the spine.

"Wind Mansion" (GV16): At the top of the spinal column in the large hollow under the base of the skull.

"Third Eye Point" (GV24.5): Directly between the eyebrows, in the indentation where the bridge of the nose meets the forehead.

"Bigger Rushing" (Lv3): On the top of the foot, in the webbing between the big toe and the second toe.

Exercises

1. Press B2. Place your thumbs on the upper ridge of your eye sockets close to the bridge of the nose. Press upward into the indentations of the eye sockets as you breath deeply for one minute.

2. Hold St2 & St3. Place your index fingers in the center of your cheeks below the lower ridge of the eyes, in line with the pupil. Then place you thumbs directly below your index fingers, underneath the cheekbones. With your eyes closed, apply light pressure and breathe deeply for a minute.

3. Press BIO. Curve your fingers to firmly press BIO on the muscles that run parallel to the spine. Hold for one minute as you breath deeply.

4. Hold GV16 and GV24.5. Place the middle finger of your left hand on GV16 in the large hollow in the middle of the base of your skull. Use the middle finger of your right hand to lightly touch GV24.5 and focus your attention on that spot with your eyes closed. Breathe deeply as you hold this powerful healing point for one minute.

5. Stimulate Lv3. Slip your shoes off. Starting between your large and second toes on both feet, slide your middle and index fingers up the foot in the valley between the bones. Press firmly into the indentation just before the bones join to form a V shape. Rub against the skin to stimulate these eyestrain relief points.

Eastern herbs

Here's a list of Eastern herbs touted as vision aids.

Xi Gan Ming Mu. Gardenia and Vitex combination. This formula contains 19 herbs that benefit eye disorders.

Zi Shen Ming Mu Tang. Chrysanthemum combination. Good for healing eye problems resulting from liver and kidney problems.

Ming Mu Shang Qing Plan. Bright Eyes Upper Clearing tablets. Sedates the liver "fire," which upsets the eyes.

Net Zhang Ming Yan Wan. Inner Obstruction to Eyesight pills. Encourages visual clarity and nourishes the liver and kidneys.

Shi Hu Ye Guang Wan. Dendrobium Leaf Night Sight pills. Nourishes the blood and tonifies the liver and kidneys. Aids blurry or dizzy sight, hypersensitivity, and intraocular pressure.

Ming Mu Di Huang Wan. Bright Eyes Rehmannia pills. Replenishes the liver and kidneys, nourishes the blood, and sedates liver "fire and wind."

The benefits of vitamin A

"Eat your carrots," our parents admonished us, "they're good for your eyes." And they were right. Carrots, and all sources of vitamin A and beta-carotene, are excellent for overall eye care.

We know that vitamin A is essential for human vision. In fact, vitamin A and its relation to eye care is one of the more studied uses for the vitamins — dating back some 50 years.

Symptoms of Vitamin A deficiency include poor rapid-dark adaptation, pink or inflamed eyelids, and dryness of the cornea. So you can see how important vitamin A is to overall vision. An effective dose (under supervision of a holistic doctor) for night blindness is 25,000 IU per day for one month with at least 25 mg of zinc per day.

There has been a lot of well-deserved press lately about the A-related nutrient, beta carotene, and its power as an antioxidant. This power extends to the eye: Beta carotene is very helpful in fighting certain chemical reactions that can lead to macular degeneration. Beta-carotene, working as an antioxidant, helps to eliminate free radicals — those free oxygen molecules that contribute to the aging process.

When you take vitamin A and when you eat vegetables containing beta carotene, your body converts the beta carotene to various forms of A called retinols. Your body uses these retinols for numerous things — repairing ligaments, transporting various enzymes, and playing a role in the bio-electrical process of vision.

In the eye, beta-carotene is converted to the aldehyde form of vitamin A. Your body uses aldehyde to initiate the electrical energy that travels along the optic nerve to the cortex of the brain — the place where vision is "created."

As our parents so often told us, a deficiency of "carrots" leads to night blindness — the inability to adapt to low-light situations. A severe shortage of vitamin A and beta carotene can indeed lead to blindness.

A specific hereditary disease, retinitis pigmentosa, causes similar symptoms in the early stages. Symptoms are related to retinal/opsin metabolic deficiency secondary to the primary degenerative pigmentary changes and resulting destruction of the photoreceptors. Treatment with massive doses of beta-carotene and vitamin A acids has been shown to be effective in the early stages of the disease. Take up to 25,000 IU of vitamin A and 10,000 IU of beta carotene per day.

Note: If you're pregnant, don't take over 10,000 IU of vitamin A. Beta carotene is much safer for the baby.

Beta-carotene relatives

Evidence continues to mount supporting the theory that at least three other carotenoids (lutein, xyline, and zeaxanthin) play a role in age-related macular degeneration (ARMD). Researchers at Harvard Medical School compared the dietary habits of patients diagnosed with ARMD to those with other eye pathologies but without ARMD. They found a direct correlation with increased consumption of carotenoids and decreased risk of ARMD.

Science has long accepted the role of beta carotene's related compounds in retinal neurological processing, but recent studies indicate that some of the other carotenoids may have more profound effects on the aging eye. Vitamin C in its many forms (acids and mineral-bound ascorbates) is also important in tissue repair and as an antioxidant. Along with the antioxidant minerals selenium, chromium, and the polypeptide glutathione (and its related amino acid glutamine), these nutrients may provide the key to maintaining better visual function in later life.

In recent years, researchers have found that the lack of a number of other common nutrients are involved in the aging of the eye. These antioxidants and key elements active in the metabolic processes include: vitamin C, vitamin E, and vitamin D. The minerals zinc, chromium, and selenium, as well as the amino acid 1-glutathione, are also involved in the process.

Does taking more of these nutrients into your body slow the aging process? There are many factors responsible for the aging of the eye (and the rest of us) and these nutrients certainly play a role. Quite a few health practitioners and nutritionists now recommend supplementation of these vitamins, minerals, and amino acids to slow the loss of vision. I have to agree.

A list of essential nutrients

Here's a brief summary of some essential nutrients and how they can help to improve the function of the eye. B group Vitamins, should be taken as a complex:

Vitamin B_1 (thiamine): is one of the most important of the B group vitamins. Symptoms B_1 deficiency include cystic breasts, burning or bloodshot eyes, unclear or double vision, conjunctivitis, eye fatigue, sensitivity to light, and dark spots in the visual field. If you have any of these symptoms, I suggest a daily dose of at least 500 mgs, which means that you cannot get the recommended dose in a multivitamin tablet as you can most of the other vitamins and minerals. So you will need to take an extra supplement. If you don't have a thiamine deficiency, 100 mgs will suffice.

Vitamin B_2 (riboflavin): Symptoms of lack of B_2 are burning or bloodshot eyes, conjunctivitis, eye fatigue, sensitivity to light, pupil dilation, twilight blindness, and dark spots in the visual field. If you suffer from a riboflavin deficiency, see a holistic doctor for dosages. Otherwise, you need to be taking at least 50 mg daily.

61

Vitamin B$_6$ may be involved in regulating eye pressure and may help prevent glaucoma. Take 100 mg daily.

Vitamin B$_{12}$: Symptoms of B$_{12}$ deficiency may include a general dimming of vision. To avoid this problem, take 100 meg daily.

Vitamin C (ascorbic acid): The sclera of the eye depends on Vitamin C, and cataracts may begin when Vitamin C becomes deficient. Glaucoma may also be treated by Vitamin C, two grams (2,000 mg) daily for six days, then reduce to the normal 1,200 mg. There is no know toxic dose. Vitamin C should be taken with bioflavinoids.

Vitamin D and Calcium are another important combination. There is evidence linking a childhood deficiency of these two to myopia. Vitamin D is needed for the assimilation of calcium, and the prevention of waterlogged sclera. If the fibrous tunic around the eye has excess water, the interocular pressure may build up leading to elongation and myopia. Vitamin D and calcium have been shown to dehydrate the water from the sclera and reduce elongation.

Optometrist Ben Lane demonstrated that myopic children tended to have a diet higher in refined carbohydrates than clear-seeing children. This results in a deficiency of minerals, vitamins, calcium, and chromium, and an overabundance of phosphorus. High phosphorus reduces calcium levels. I suggest you get 400 IU of vitamin D and 500 mg of calcium each day.

Vitamin E has been shown to have a positive effect on some types of eye pathology. I suggest a dose of a least 400 units of vitamin E daily.

Zinc: Dark adaptation may be impaired by zinc deficiency. Taken in conjunction with vitamin A, it has been shown to alleviate macular degeneration and poor night vision. Make sure that supplemental zinc (25-100 mg) is mixed with copper (2 mg) and selenium (200 meg) — check your multi formula for these minerals.

Chromium is vital for bodily regulation of energy. Deficiencies are caused by excess sugar in the diet. A good dose is 200 meg/day.

Lutein (mentioned earlier) is just now becoming available in tablet form. If you can find lutein tablets, I suggest that you use these tablets at the dosage recommend by your holistic doctor. This is particularly important for older Americans who may be experiencing the beginnings of macular degeneration. I also suggest you take 25-100 mg of **1-glutathione.**

Some eye diseases require greater doses of certain nutrients than I've listed here. These have been listed in this manuscript under the corresponding problem.

Bilberry

Bilberry, and its related plants like blueberry, has been used by the Chinese for centuries as a digestive aid, as a stimulant to the circulatory system, and as a way to improve vision. Our pioneer ancestors used blueberry to treat diabetes.

Scientific research tells us that bilberry contains many interesting chemicals, including ericolin, arbutin, beta-amyrin, nonacosane, and anthocyanosides. Anthocyanosides, which cause the deep blue-red color of many berries, seems to protect the vascular system by strengthening the capillary walls. This attribute may produce many of the secondary benefits, such as lowering of blood pressure, reduction of clots, reducing varicosities and bruising, reversing poor circulation, and thus improving blood supply to tissues.

As researcher Robert Bidleman reports, bilberry is used in Europe before surgery to prevent excessive bleeding and hemorrhaging. A recent German medical journal reports bilberry effective in reducing bleeding tendencies by 71 percent. Bilberry also thins the blood by inhibiting platelet adhesion. This combination of actions — improving capillary strength, reduction of capillary leakage, and blood thinning — results in improved blood flow and may reduce clotting-related health risks.

But when it comes to helping vision, bilberry seems nothing short of amazing. During World War II, Royal Air Force (RAF) pilots were forced to fly at night. Many pilots and their crew members complained of the poor visibility and its effects on their performance. But, the pilots noticed that if they ate bilberry jam, their night vision improved.

Some years later, researched discovered what the pilots already knew: Bilberry's powerful effects increased retinal purple (rhodopsin) by dramatic amounts in just 20 minutes, sometimes less. One study showed bilberry to improve eyesight and increase ocular blood supply in 75 percent of patients. It improved near-sightedness after five months of regular use, while an 83 percent improvement in visual acuity was recorded after only 15 days.

One of the more encouraging statistics regarding bilberry's visual-enhancing properties is that over 80 percent of the people taking bilberry for the first time improved on their visual acuity exam and passed a night-vision test. Long-term improvements took an average of six weeks with regular doses.

Add to this, bilberry's known antioxidant effects — more powerful than vitamins E and C — and it's easy to see why bilberry is an ideal herb for the overall care of your eyes.

As a bonus, if you're having digestive problems, taking bilberry for your eyes may also help settle your stomach.

While bilberry is available in many forms, the most powerful is concentrated extract. If you decide to try bilberry, I suggest this form. And follow the manufacturers recommended dosage.

Along with bilberry, "eyebright" is another herb that can help your vision. Eyebright is a native herb of Europe with a long history of use in vision. Recommended for eye inflammations, stinging or weeping eyes, and hypersensitivity to light. Please see page 37 for the recipe of an excellent eyewash with this and other herbs.

As you can see, there are a number of things you can try to use to improve your eyesight. Of course, not everything will work in every case, but many are harmless. So go ahead a try them, and let me know what worked for you.

About Doctor William Campbell Douglass II

Dr. Douglass reveals medical truths, and deceptions, often at risk of being labeled heretical. He is consumed by a passion for living a long healthy life, and wants his readers to share that passion. Their health and well-being comes first. He is anti-dogmatic, and unwavering in his dedication to improve the quality of life of his readers. He has been called "the conscience of modern medicine," a "medical maverick," and has been voted "Doctor of the Year" by the National Health Federation. His medical experiences are far reaching-from battling malaria in Central America - to fighting deadly epidemics at his own health clinic in Africa - to flying with U.S. Navy crews as a flight surgeon - to working for 10 years in emergency medicine here in the States. These learning experiences, not to mention his keen storytelling ability and wit, make Dr. Douglass' newsletters (Daily Dose and Real Health) and books uniquely interesting and fun to read. He shares his no-frills, no-bull approach to health care, often amazing his readers by telling them to ignore many widely-hyped good-health practices (like staying away from red meat, avoiding coffee, and eating like a bird), and start living again by eating REAL food, taking some inexpensive supplements, and doing the pleasurable things that make life livable. Readers get all this, plus they learn how to burn fat, prevent cancer, boost libido, and so much more. And, Dr. Douglass is not afraid to challenge the latest studies that come out, and share the real story with his readers. Dr. William C. Douglass has led a colorful, rebellious, and crusading life. Not many physicians would dare put their professional reputations on the line as many times as this courageous healer has. A vocal opponent of "business-as-usual" medicine, Dr. Douglass has championed patients' rights and physician commitment to wellness throughout his career. This dedicated physician has repeatedly gone far beyond the call of duty in his work to spread the truth about alternative therapies. For a full year, he endured economic and physical hardship to work with physicians at the Pasteur Institute in St. Petersburg, Russia, where advanced research on photoluminescence was being conducted. Dr. Douglass comes from a distinguished family of physicians. He is the fourth generation Douglass to practice medicine, and his son is also a physician. Dr. Douglass graduated from the University of Rochester, the Miami School of Medicine, and the Naval School of Aviation and Space Medicine.

You want to protect those you love from the health dangers the authorities aren't telling you about, and learn the incredible cures that they've scorned and ignored?

Subscribe to the free Daily Dose updates "...the straight scoop about health, medicine, and politics." by sending an e-mail to real_sub@agoramail.net with the word "subscribe" in the subject line.

Dr. William Campbell Douglass'
Real Health:

Had Enough?

Enough turkey burgers and sprouts?

Enough forcing gallons of water down your throat?

Enough exercising until you can barely breathe?

Before you give up everything just because "everyone" says it's healthy...

Learn the facts from Dr. William Campbell Douglass, medicine's most acclaimed myth-buster. In every issue of Dr. Douglass' Real Health newsletter, you'll learn shocking truths about "junk medicine" and how to stay healthy while eating eggs, meat and other foods you love.

With the tips you'll receive from Real Health, you'll see your doctor less, spend a lot less money and be happier and healthier while you're at it. The road to Real Health is actually easier, cheaper and more pleasant than you dared to dream.

Subscribe to Real Health today by calling 1-800-981-7162 or visit the Real Health web site at www.realhealthnews.com.
Use promotional code : DRHBDZZZ

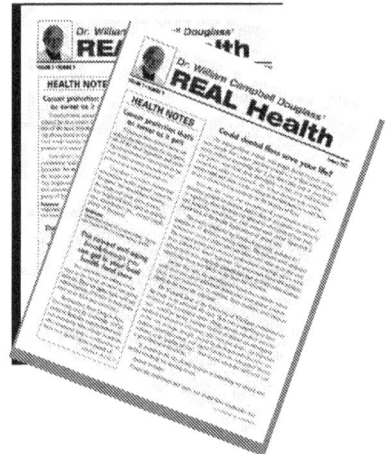

If you knew of a procedure that could save thousands, maybe millions, of people dying from AIDS, cancer, and other dreaded killers....

Would you cover it up?

It's unthinkable that what could be the best solution ever to stopping the world's killer diseases is being ignored, scorned, and rejected. But that is exactly what's happening right now.

The procedure is called "photoluminescence". It's a thoroughly tested, proven therapy that uses the healing power of the light to perform almost miraculous cures.

This remarkable treatment works its incredible cures by stimulating the body's own immune responses. That's why it cures so many ailments--and why it's been especially effective against AIDS! Yet, 50 years ago, it virtually disappeared from the halls of medicine.

Why has this incredible cure been ignored by the medical authorities of this country? You'll find the shocking answer here in the pages of this new edition of Into the Light. Now available with the blood irradiation Instrument Diagram and a complete set of instructions for building your own "Treatment Device". Also includes details on how to use this unique medical instrument.

Into the Light

Into the Light

Rhino Publishing S.A.
www.rhinopublish.com

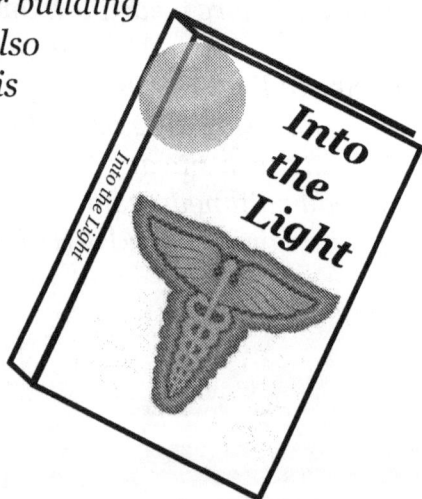

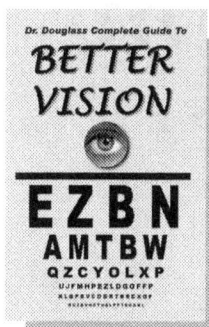

Dr. Douglass' Complete Guide to Better Vision

A report about eyesight and what can be done to improve it naturally. But I've also included information about how the eye works, brief descriptions of various common eye conditions, traditional remedies to eye problems, and a few simple suggestions that may help you maintain your eyesight for years to come.
-William Campbell Douglass II, MD

The Hypertension Report.
Say Good Bye to High Blood Pressure.

An estimated 50 million Americans have high blood pressure. Often called the "silent killer" because it may not cause symptoms until the patient has suffered serious damage to the arterial system. Diet, exercise, potassium supplements chelation therapy and practically anything but drugs is the way to go and alternatives are discussed in this report.

Grandma Bell's A To Z Guide To Healing With Herbs.

This book is all about - coming home. What I once believed to be old wives' tales - stories long destroyed by the new world of science - actually proved to be the best treatment for many of the common ailments you and I suffer through. So I put a few of them together in this book with the sincere hope that Grandma Bell's wisdom will help you recover your common sense, and take responsibility for your own health. -William Campbell Douglass II, MD

Prostate Problems:
Safe, Simple, Effective Relief for Men over 50.

Don't be frightened into surgery or drugs you may not need. First, get the facts about prostate problems... know all your options, so you can make the best decisions. This fully documented report explains the dangers of conventional treatments, and gives you alternatives that could save you more than just money!

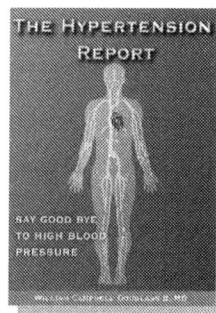

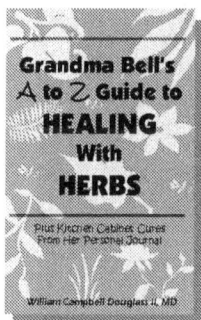

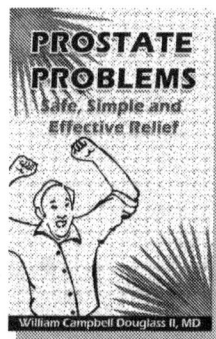

Color me Healthy
The Healing Powers of Colors

"He's crazy!"
"He's got to be a quack!"
"Who gave this guy his medical license?"
"He's a nut case!"

In case you're wondering, those are the reactions you'll probably get if you show your doctor this report. I know the idea of healing many common ailments simply by exposing them to colored light sounds far-fetched, but when you see the evidence, you'll agree that color is truly an amazing medical breakthrough.

When I first heard the stories, I reacted much the same way. But the evidence so convinced me, that I had to try color therapy in my practice. My results were truly amazing.

-William Campbell Douglass II, MD

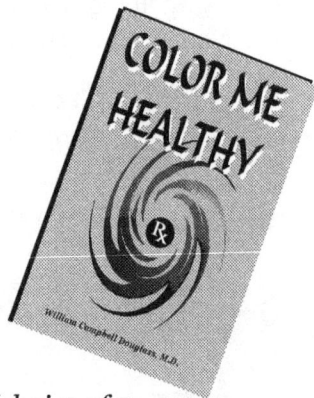

Order your complete set of Roscolene filters (choice of 3 sizes) to be used with the "Color Me Healthy" therapy. The eleven Roscolene filters are # 809, 810, 818, 826, 828, 832, 859, 861, 866, 871, and 877. The filters come with protective separator sheets between each filter. The color names and the Roscolene filter(s) used to produce that particular color, are printed on a card included with the filters and a set of instructions on how to fit them to a lamp.

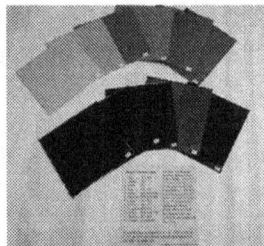

Rhino Publishing
www.rhinopublish.com

What Is Going on Here?

Peroxides are supposed to be bad for you. Free radicals and all that. But now we hear that hydrogen peroxide is good for us. Hydrogen peroxide will put extra oxygen in your blood. There's no doubt about that. Hydrogen peroxide costs pennies. So if you can get oxygen into the blood cheaply and safely, maybe cancer (which doesn't like oxygen), emphysema, AIDS, and many other terrible diseases can be treated effectively. Intravenous hydrogen peroxide rapidly relieves allergic reactions, influenza symptoms, and acute viral infections.

No one expects to live forever. But we would all like to have a George Burns finish. The prospect of finishing life in a nursing home after abandoning your tricycle in the mobile home park is not appealing. Then comes the loss of control of vital functions the ultimate humiliation. Is life supposed to be from tricycle to tricycle and diaper to diaper? You come into this world crying, but do you have to leave crying? I don't believe you do. And you won't either after you see the evidence. Sounds too good to be true, doesn't it? Read on and decide for yourself.

-William Campbell Douglass II, MD

Rhino Publishing S.A.
www.rhinopublish.com

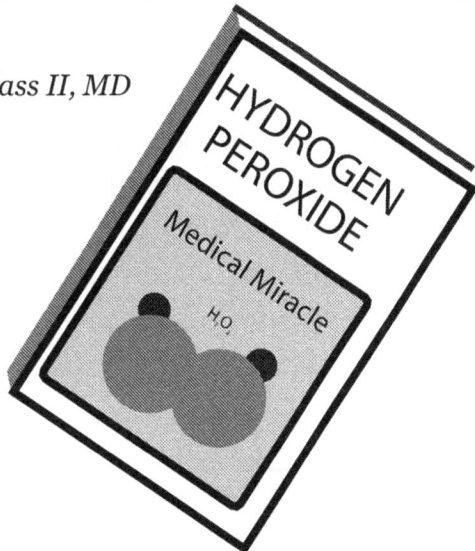

HYDROGEN PEROXIDE

Medical Miracle

H_2O_2

Don't drink your milk!

If you knew what we know about milk... BLEECHT! All that pasteurization, homogenization and processing is not only cooking all the nutrients right out of your favorite drink. It's also adding toxic levels of vitamin D.

This fascinating book tells the whole story about milk. How it once was nature's perfect food...how "raw," unprocessed milk can heal and boost your immune system ... why you can't buy it legally in this country anymore, and what we could do to change that.

Dr. "Douglass traveled all over the world, tasting all kinds of milk from all kinds of cows, poring over dusty research books in ancient libraries far from home, to write this light-hearted but scientifically sound book.

Rhino Publishing, S.A.
www.rhinopublish.com

The Milk Book

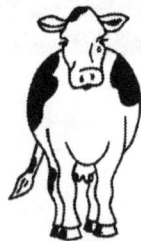

William Campbell Douglass II, MD

Eat Your Cholesterol!
Eat Meat, Drink Milk, Spread The Butter- And Live Longer!
How to Live off the Fat of the Land and Feel Great.

Americans are being saturated with anti-cholesterol propaganda. If you watch very much television, you're probably one of the millions of Americans who now has a terminal case of cholesterol phobia. The propaganda is relentless and is often designed to produce fear and loathing of this worst of all food contaminants. You never hear the food propagandists bragging about their product being fluoride-free or aluminum-free, two of our truly serious food-additive problems. But cholesterol, an essential nutrient, not proven to be harmful in any quantity, is constantly pilloried as a menace to your health. If you don't use corn oil, Fleischmann's margarine, and Egg Beaters, you're going straight to atherosclerosis hell with stroke, heart attack, and premature aging -- and so are your kids. Never feel guilty about what you eat again! Dr. Douglass shows you why red meat, eggs, and dairy products aren't the dietary demons we're told they are. But beware: This scientifically sound report goes against all the "common wisdom" about the foods you should eat. Read with an open mind.

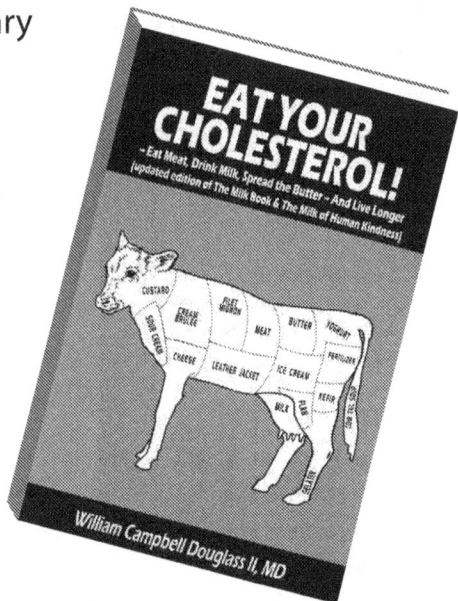

EAT YOUR CHOLESTEROL!
- Eat Meat, Drink Milk, Spread the Butter - And Live Longer
(updated edition of The Milk Book & The Milk of Human Kindness)

CUSTARD
CREAM BRULEE
SOUR CREAM
FILET MIGNON
MEAT
BUTTER
YOGHURT
PORRIDGE
CHEESE
LEATHER JACKET
ICE CREAM
MILK
EGG

William Campbell Douglass II, MD

Rhino Publishing, S.A.
www.rhinopublish.com

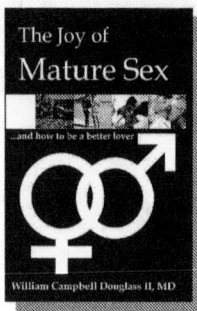

The Joy of Mature Sex and How to Be a Better Lover

Humans are very confused about what makes good sex. But I believe humans have more to offer each other than this total licentiousness common among animals. We're talking about mature sex. The kind of sex that made this country great.

Stop Aging or Slow the Process How Exercise With Oxygen Therapy (EWOT) Can Help

EWOT (pronounced ee-watt) stands for Exercise With Oxygen Therapy. This method of prolonging your life is so simple and you can do it at home at a minimal cost. When your cells don't get enough oxygen, they degenerate and die and so you degenerate and die. It's as simple as that.

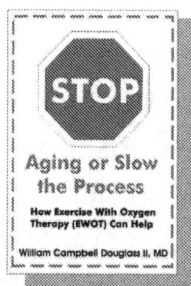

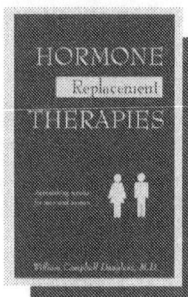

Hormone Replacement Therapies: Astonishing Results For Men And Women

It is accurate to say that when the endocrine glands start to fail, you start to die. We are facing a sea change in longevity and health in the elderly. Now, with the proper supplemental hormones, we can slow the aging process and, in many cases, reverse some of the signs and symptoms of aging.

Add 10 Years to Your Life With some "best of" Dr. Douglass' writings.

To add ten years to your life, you need to have the right attitude about health and an understanding of the health industry and what it's feeding you. Following the established line on many health issues could make you very sick or worse! Achieve dynamic health with this collection of some of the "best of" Dr. Douglass' newsletters.

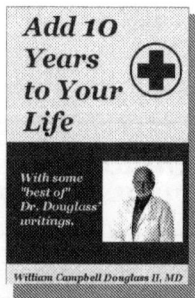

How did AIDS become one of the Greatest Biological Disasters in the History of Mankind?

GET THE FACTS

AIDS and BIOLOGICAL WARFARE covers the history of plagues from the past to today's global confrontation with AIDS, the Prince of Plagues. Completely documented *AIDS and BIOLOGICAL WARFARE* helps you make your own decisions about how to survive in a world ravaged by this horrible plague.

You will learn that AIDS is not a naturally occuring disease process as you have been led to believe, but a man-made biological nightmare that has been unleashed and is now threatening the very existence of human life on the planet.

There is a smokescreen of misinformation clouding the AIDS issue. Now, for the first time, learn the truth about the nature of the crisis our planet faces: its origin -- how AIDS is really transmited and alternatives for treatment. Find out what they are not telling you about AIDS and Biological Warfare, and how to protect yourself and your loved ones. AIDS is a serious problem worldwide, but it is no longer the major threat. You need to know the whole story. To protect yourself, you must know the truth about biological warfare.

Rhino Publishing S.A.
www.rhinopublish.com

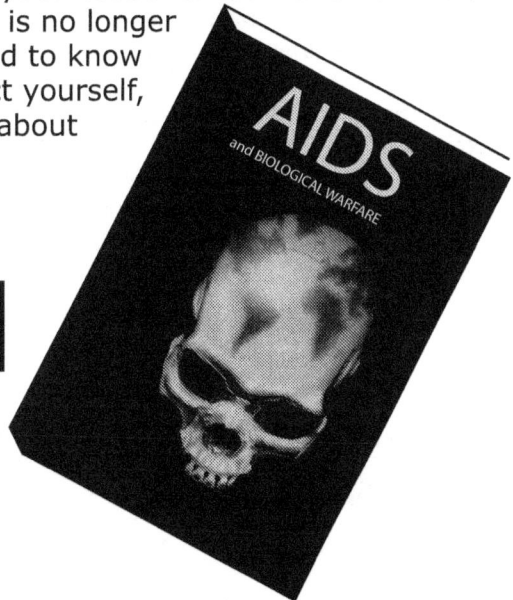

PAINFUL DILEMMA

Are we fighting the wrong war?

We are spending millions on the war against drugs while we
should be fighting the war against pain with those drugs!

As you will read in this book, the war on drugs was lost a long time ago and,
when it comes to the war against pain, pain is winning! An article in USA Today
(11/20/02) reveals that dying patients are not getting relief from pain. It seems
the doctors are torn between fear of the government, certainly justified, and a
clinging to old and out dated ideas about pain, which is NOT justified.

A group called Last Acts, a coalition of health-care groups, has released a very
discouraging study of all 50 states that nearly half of the 1.6 million Americans
living in nursing homes suffer from untreated pain. They said that life was being
extended but it amounted to little more than "extended pain and suffering."

This book offers insight into the history of pain treatment and the current failed
philosophies of contemporary medicine. Plus it describes some of today's most
advanced treatments for alleviating certain kinds of pain. This book is not another
"self-help" book touting home remedies; rather, Painful Dilemma: Patients in
Pain -- People in Prison, takes a hard look at where we've gone wrong and what
we (you) can do to help a loved one who is living with chronic pain.

The second half of this book is a must read if you value your freedom. We now
have the ridiculous and tragic situation of people
in pain living in a government-created hell by
restriction of narcotics and people in prison for
trying to bring pain relief by the selling of
narcotics to the suffering. The end result of the
"war on drugs" has been to create the greatest
and most destructive cartel in history, so great,
in fact, that the drug Mafia now controls most
of the world economy.

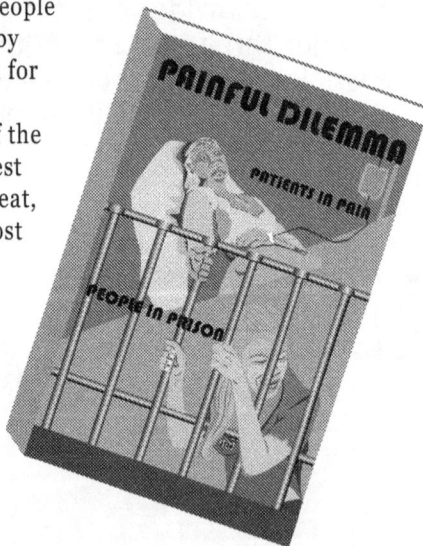

Rhino Publishing S.A.
www.rhinopublish.com

Live the Adventure!

Why would anyone in their right mind put everything they own in storage and move to Russia, of all places?! But when maverick physician Bill Douglass left a profitable medical practice in a peaceful mountaintop town to pursue "pure medical truth".... none of us who know him well was really surprised.

After All, anyone who's braved the outermost reaches of darkest Africa, the mean streets of Johannesburg and New York, and even a trip to Washington to testify before the Senate, wouldn't bat and eye at ducking behind the Iron Curtain for a little medical reconnaissance!

Enjoy this imaginative, funny, dedicated man's tales of wonder and woe as he treks through a year in St. Petersburg, working on a cure for the world's killer diseases. We promise --

YOU WON'T BE BORED!

Rhino Publishing S.A.
www.rhinopublish.com

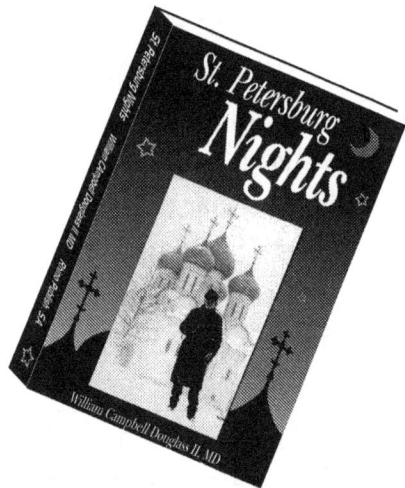

St. Petersburg Nights

William Campbell Douglass II MD

THE SMOKER'S PARADOX
THE HEALTH BENEFITS OF TOBACCO!

The benefits of smoking tobacco have been common knowledge for centuries. From sharpening mental acuity to maintaining optimal weight, the relatively small risks of smoking have always been outweighed by the substantial improvement to mental and physical health. Hysterical attacks on tobacco notwithstanding, smokers always weigh the good against the bad and puff away or quit according to their personal preferences. Now the same anti-tobacco enterprise that has spent billions demonizing the pleasure of smoking is providing additional reasons to smoke. Alzheimer's, Parkinson's, Tourette's Syndrome, even schizophrenia and cocaine addiction are disorders that are alleviated by tobacco. Add in the still inconclusive indication that tobacco helps to prevent colon and prostate cancer and the endorsement for smoking tobacco by the medical establishment is good news for smokers and non-smokers alike. Of course the revelation that tobacco is good for you is ruined by the pharmaceutical industry's plan to substitute the natural and relatively inexpensive tobacco plant with their overpriced and ineffective nicotine substitutions. Still, when all is said and done, the positive revelations regarding tobacco are very good reasons indeed to keep lighting those cigars - but only 4 a day!

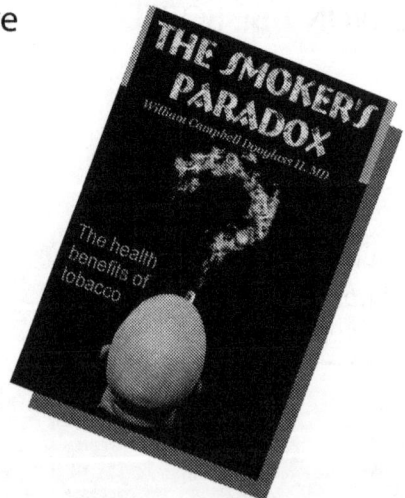

Rhino Publishing, S.A
www.rhinopublish.com

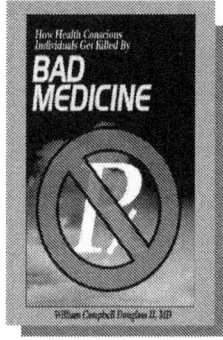

Bad Medicine
How Individuals Get Killed By Bad Medicine.

Do you really need that new prescription or that overnight stay in the hospital? In this report, Dr. Douglass reveals the common medical practices and misconceptions endangering your health. Best of all, he tells you the pointed (but very revealing!) questions your doctor prays you never ask. Interesting medical facts about popular remedies are revealed.

Dangerous Legal Drugs
The Poisons in Your Medicine Chest.

If you knew what we know about the most popular prescription and over-the-counter drugs, you'd be sick. That's why Dr. Douglass wrote this shocking report about the poisons in your medicine chest. He gives you the low-down on different categories of drugs. Everything from painkillers and cold remedies to tranquilizers and powerful cancer drugs.

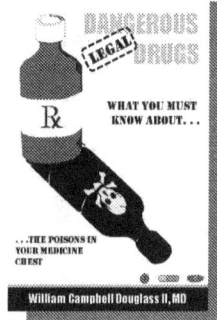

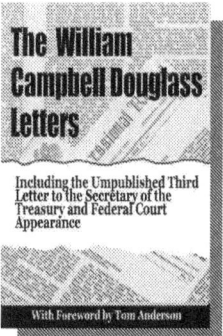

The William Campbell Douglass Letters.
Expose of Government Machinations (Vietnam War).

THE WILLIAM CAMPBELL DOUGLASS LETTERS. Dr. Douglass' Defense in 1968 Tax Case and Expose of Government Machinations during the Vietnam War.

The Eagle's Feather. A Novel of International Political Intrigue.

Although The Eagle's Feather is a work of fiction set in the 1970's, it is built, as with most fiction, on a framework of plausibility and background information. This is a fiction book that could not have been written were it not for various ominous aspects, which pose a clear and present danger to the security of the United States.

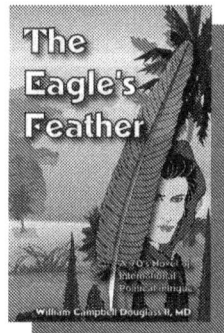

Rhino Publishing

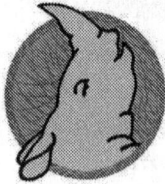

ORDER FORM

PURCHASER INFORMATION

Purchaser's Name (Please Print): _____

Shipping Address (Do not use a P.O. Box): _____

City: _____ State/Prov.: _____ Country: _____

Zip/Postal Code: _____ Telephone No.: _____ Fax No.: _____

E-Mail Address (if interested in receiving free e-Books when available): _____

CREDIT CARD INFO (CIRCLE ONE):

MASTERCARD, VISA, AMERICAN EXPRESS, DISCOVER, JCB, DINER'S CLUB, CARTE BLANCHE.

Charge my Card -> Number #: _____ Exp.: _____

*Security Code: _____ * Required for all MasterCard, Visa and American Express purchases. For your security, we require that you enter your card's verification number. The verification number is also called a CCV number. This code is the 3 digits farthest right in the signature field on the back of your VISA/MC, or the 4 digits to the right on the front of your American Express card. Your credit card statement will show **a different name than Rhino Publishing** as the vendor.

WE DO NOT share your private information, we use 3rd party credit card processing service to process your order only.

ADDITIONAL INFORMATION

If your shipping address is not the same as your credit card billing address, please indicate your card billing address here.

Name on the card _____   Type of card: _____

Billing Address: _____

City: _____   State/Prov.: _____   Zip/Postal Code: _____

Fax a copy of this order to:
RHINO PUBLISHING, S.A.
1-888-317-6767 or International #: + 416-352-5126

To order by mail, send your payment by first class mail only to the following address. Please include a copy of this order form. Make your check or bank drafts (NO postal money order) payable to RHINO PUBLISHING, S.A. and mail to:

Rhino Publishing, S.A.
Attention: PTY 5048
P.O. Box 025724
Miami, FL.
USA 33102

Digital E-books also available online: www.rhinopublish.com

Rhino Publishing

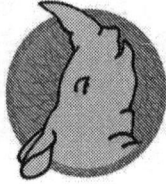

ORDER FORM

Purchaser's Name (Please Print): _____

I would like to order the following paperback book of Dr. Douglass (Alternative Medicine Books):

___	X	9962-636-04-3	Add 10 Years to Your Life. With some "best of" Dr. Douglass writings.	$13.99 $ _____
___	X	9962-636-07-8	AIDS and Biological Warfare. What They Are Not Telling You!	$17.99 $ _____
___	X	9962-636-09-4	Bad Medicine. How Individuals Get Killed By Bad Medicine.	$11.99 $ _____
___	X	9962-636-10-8	Color Me Healthy. The Healing Power of Colors.	$11.99 $ _____
___	X	9962-636 -XX-X	Color Filters for Color Me Healthy. 11 Basic Roscolene Filters for Lamps.	$21.89 $ _____
___	X	9962-636-15-9	Dangerous Legal Drugs. The Poisons in Your Medicine Chest.	$13.99 $ _____
___	X	9962-636-18-3	Dr. Douglass' Complete Guide to Better Vision. Improve eyesight naturally.	$11.99 $ _____
___	X	9962-636-19-1	Eat Your Cholesterol! How to Live off the Fat of the Land and Feel Great.	$11.99 $ _____
___	X	9962-636-12-4	Grandma Bell's A To Z Guide To Healing. Her Kitchen Cabinet Cures.	$14.99 $ _____
___	X	9962-636-22-1	Hormone Replacement Therapies. Astonishing Results For Men & Women	$11.99 $ _____
___	X	9962-636-25-6	Hydrogen Peroxide: One of the Most Underused Medical Miracle.	$15.99 $ _____
___	X	9962-636-27-2	Into the Light. New Edition with Blood Irradiation Instrument Instructions.	$19.99 $ _____
___	X	9962-636-54-X	Milk Book. The Classic on the Nutrition of Milk and How to Benefit from it.	$17.99 $ _____

___	X	9962-636-00-0	Painful Dilemma - Patients in Pain - People in Prison.	$17.99	$___
___	X	9962-636-32-9	Prostate Problems. Safe, Simple, Effective Relief for Men over 50.	$11.99	$___
___	X	9962-636-34-5	St. Petersburg Nights. Enlightening Story of Life and Science in Russia.	$17.99	$___
___	X	9962-636-37-X	Stop Aging or Slow the Process. Exercise With Oxygen Therapy Can Help.	$11.99	$___
___	X	9962-636-60-4	The Hypertension Report. Say Good Bye to High Blood Pressure.	$11.99	$___
___	X	9962-636-48-5	The Joy of Mature Sex and How to Be a Better Lover...	$13.99	$___
___	X	9962-636-43-4	The Smoker's Paradox: Health Benefits of Tobacco.	$14.99	$___

Political Books:

___	X	9962-636-40-X	The Eagle's Feather. A 70's Novel of International Political Intrigue.	$15.99	$___
___	X	9962-636-46-9	The W. C. D. Letters. Expose of Government Machinations (Vietnam War).	$11.99	$___

SUB-TOTAL: $___

ADD $5.00 HANDLING FOR YOUR ORDER: $ 5.00 $ 5.00

___ X ADD $2.50 SHIPPING FOR EACH ITEM ON ORDER: $ 2.50 $___

NOTE THAT THE MINIMUM SHIPPING AND HANDLING IS $7.50 FOR 1 BOOK ($5.00 + $2.50)
For order shipped outside the US, add $5.00 per item

___ X ADD $5.00 S. & H. OR EACH ITEM ON ORDER (INTERNATIONAL ORDERS ONLY) $ 5.00 $___
Allow up to 21 days for delivery (we will call you about back orders if any)

TOTAL: $___

Fax a copy of this order to: 1-888-317-6767 or Int'l + 416-352-5126
or mail to: Rhino Publishing, S.A. Attention: PTY 5048 P.O. Box 025724, Miami, FL., 33102 USA
Digital E-books also available online: www.rhinopublish.com

www.ingramcontent.com/pod-product-compliance
Lightning Source LLC
Chambersburg PA
CBHW032102020426
42335CB00011B/459